Dash Diet for Weight Loss

Your Dash Diet Cookbook and Guide to Lose Weight Fast, Lower Blood Pressure and Live a Healthy Life!

Introduction

I want to thank you and congratulate you for buying the book, *"Dash Diet for Weight Loss - Your Dash Diet Cookbook and Guide to Lose Weight Fast, Lower Blood Pressure and Live a Healthy Life!"*

I think we all agree that losing weight is quite challenging. I mean, with some weight loss diets requiring you to only take smoothies for a while, others using juices only and others no carbohydrates, losing weight can be quite complicated. However, although losing weight and living a healthy life is indeed challenging, you can still achieve your goals without necessarily having to starve yourself or greatly reducing the amount of calories you eat. With the DASH diet, you can lower your blood pressure, lose weight and live a healthy life. This book will help you to understand what the DASH diet is, how it works and gives some recipes to get started on the DASH diet. Actually, the book has over 40 DASH diet recipes written just for you.

In the first chapter of this book, I have given an overview of the diet. This section will answer all your preliminary questions about this diet. In the second chapter, I have highlighted the principles of the diet, which will help you appreciate the nuances of this diet. In the third chapter of this book, I have highlighted how effective the DASH diet is, when it comes to improving our health. To help you get a clear picture of what this diet exactly prescribes, I have given a sample diet chart in the fourth chapter. This should help you plan your diet chart accordingly. As a new dieter, you might be frantic about following the diet. To put you out of your misery, I have given some tips in the fifth chapter.

These tips cover a whole range of topics, starting from shopping till dining out. The last four chapters are exclusively dedicated for recipes. I am sure that these mouthwatering recipes will definitely excite you and motivate you to get started as soon as possible.

I am sure that you will definitely appreciate how the DASH diet is instrumental in helping you lead a healthy lifestyle, by the end of this book.

Thanks again for buying this book and I hope you enjoy it!

information is without contract or any type of guarantee assurance.

The trademarks that are used are without any consent, and the publication of the trademark is without permission or backing by the trademark owner. All trademarks and brands within this book are for clarifying purposes only and are the owned by the owners themselves, not affiliated with this document.

Table of Contents

Chapter 1: DASH Diet – An Overview

I am sure that I have caught your attention, when it comes to the DASH diet. It is important that you know what the DASH diet is all about. Only when you understand what goes into the diet, will you be able to appreciate the effectiveness and the superiority of this diet when compared with the other diets in the market. Hence, in this chapter, you will find answers to all the preliminary questions you might have about the diet.

What is the DASH diet?

The DASH (Dietary Approaches to Stop Hypertension) diet was designed by the National Heart, Lung and Blood Institute, U.S.A, with a view to prevent as well as control hypertension through diet. It is typically a diet that needs to be adopted for lifetime and not something that you just experiment for a few weeks, if you are keen on staying away from hypertension. This diet aims at regulating your intake of sodium. It also encourages the consumption of a variety of foods that are loaded with nutrients such as magnesium, calcium and potassium, which are capable of lowering blood pressure.

In other words, the characteristics of the DASH diet are as follows:

- ✓ It is low in cholesterol, saturated fat and total fat.
- ✓ It does not include as much red meats or sweets or foods with added sugar such as the typical American diet.

✓ It encourages the consumption of beans, legumes, fruits, vegetables, whole grains, poultry, nuts and fish in large quantities.

Even though the primary objectives of this diet are only prevention and control of hypertension, it invariably helps you lose the extra pounds you have gained over the years.

Are there any variations of the DASH diet?

Yes, there are two types of DASH diet. As we already know, the DASH diet reduces the intake of sodium. Based on the restriction on the amount of sodium to be consumed in a day, there are two variations of the DASH diet, such as:

➢ Standard DASH diet:
  This diet permits you to consume about 2300 mg of sodium on a daily basis.
➢ Lower sodium DASH diet:
  As the name suggests, this is more restrictive in nature, when it comes to the consumption of sodium. You are permitted to consume only 1,500 mg of sodium on a daily basis.

As you can see, both versions are effective in restricting the consumption of sodium. Research shows that we consume at least 3,500 mg of sodium on a daily basis. This increased intake of sodium is perhaps the reason why this generation is at a higher risk of getting hypertension, as opposed to our ancestors. The standard DASH diet can be followed by anyone. The lower sodium DASH diet is ideal for people who are 51 or older than that and people who suffer from diabetes, hypertension or chronic kidney diseases. To understand the appropriate intake of sodium every day, you should consult with your doctor.

What to eat?

Both the variations of the DASH diet prescribe the consumption of large quantities of fruits, whole grains, low fat dairy products and vegetables. It also allows you to include legumes, poultry and fish as well, but in moderate quantities. Consumption of sweets, fats and red meats are permitted, so long as you consume them in smaller quantities. As you can see, the DASH diet is low in cholesterol, fat and saturated fat.

Let us look at the ideal components of the DASH diet. These foodstuffs will help you meet the required intake of 2,000 calories a day.

Grains:

No. of servings: 6 to 8 a day.

Grains include rice, cereals, bread and pasta. Some pointers to be borne in mind, while choosing grains are as follows:

> Ensure that you include more of whole grains, as opposed to refined grains. This is because whole grains are packed with more nutrients and fiber, when compared with refined grains. Make sure that you pick products that are labeled "100% whole grain" or "100% whole wheat". So, choose whole wheat pasta instead of regular pasta. Go for brown rice instead of white rice. Choose whole grain bread or wheat bread, instead of white bread.

> Since grains are ideally low in fat, eat them as is. Do not include cream or butter or cheese sauces, while preparing your grains. These tend to naturally increase the fat content of your dish.

Vegetables:

No. of servings: 4 to 5 a day.

Vegetables are packed with fiber, minerals such as magnesium, potassium and vitamins. Include large amounts of vegetables such as carrots, tomatoes, broccoli, greens, sweet potatoes etc. Some pointers to be borne in mind, while including vegetables are as follows:

> You can opt for either fresh or frozen vegetables. When you are buying canned or frozen vegetables, make sure you choose only those, which are labeled "without added salt" or "low sodium".
> Most of us tend to include vegetables only as sides in our meal. You may want to relook at how you are including vegetables in your meal. There are exciting recipes that feature vegetables as the hero.

Fruits:

No. of servings: 4 to 5 a day.

Fruits are the easiest, when it comes to preparing them. All you need is a few minutes to whip up an amazing fruit snack. Hence, ensure that you include as much fruits as possible. Like vegetables, fruits are also packed with fiber, magnesium and potassium. Fruits are typically low in fat, except avocadoes and coconuts.

Here a few pointers, when it comes to including fruits in your diet:

> Include fruits as part of every meal. Over and above this, you may consume fruits in the form of snacks.
> Do not discard edible peels from your dish. The peels of fruits such as apples, pears and fruits that contain

pits have a different texture and can be an interesting element in your dish. These peels are also packed with fiber and nutrients.

> If you are under medication, ensure that you check with your doctor about the inclusion of citrus fruits. This is because these fruits tend to interact with the medicines that you are consuming and it may have an adverse effect on your health.

> If you are opting for canned juice or fruits, check the labels to ensure that they do not contain added sugar.

Dairy products:

No. of servings: 2 to 3 a day.

You can include dairy products such as yogurt, cheese, milk etc, for they are rich in calcium, protein and Vitamin D.

Some pointers that need to be borne in mind while including dairy products in your diet are as follows:

> Ensure that you choose only those dairy products that are low in fat or fat free. This is because most dairy products contain high amounts of saturated fat.

> You can meet your daily requirement of dairy foods by eating lots of low fat or fat free yogurt.

> It is not uncommon if some people find it difficult to digest dairy products. If that is the case, you may choose lactose free products. Alternatively, you may buy dairy products over the counter, which are capable of preventing the occurrence of lactose intolerance because of the presence of the enzyme lactase.

> Even though you can get fat free cheeses from the market, make sure that you don't consume them in

large quantities. This is because these cheeses are typically loaded with sodium.

Poultry, lean meat and fish:

No. of servings: Up to 6 a day.

Meat is a rich source of vitamins, iron, zinc and protein. Ensure that you don't consume large quantities of meat, for even lean cuts contain cholesterol and fat. Here a few things to be borne in mind, while choosing meat for your meal:

> ➤ Ensure that you trim away the skin and fat from the poultry and meat before you cook them.
> ➤ Make sure you bake or broil or grill your meat instead of frying it deeply or in fat.
> ➤ When you choose your fish, ensure that you choose those that are good for the heart such as the herring, salmon and tuna. They contain omega 3 fatty acids in large quantities, which is good for the heart and are capable of lowering your cholesterol levels.

Seeds, nuts and legumes:

No. of servings: 4 to 5 a week

You can include sunflower seeds, almonds, peas, lentils, kidney beans etc. as part of your meal. These foods are rich in terms of nutrients such as magnesium and potassium and protein. They are also packed with fiber and phytochemicals. Phytochemicals are nothing but plant compounds, which are capable of protecting you against cardiovascular diseases and cancers. Make sure that your servings are small.

Some pointers to be borne in mind while including nuts, legumes and seeds as part of your diet are as follows:

- Even though nuts have high fat content, you can include them as part of your diet, for they contain monounsaturated fats, which are healthy in nature. Nuts also contain omega 3 fatty acids. However, nuts are full of calories. Hence, make sure that you consume them only in moderate quantities.
- You can use soy based products such as tempeh and tofu. These are effective alternatives to meat as they are packed with proteins.

Fats and oils:

No. of servings: 2 to 3 a day

Consumption of fats is essential for they are instrumental in absorbing the vitamins and improving your immune system as well. However, excess consumption of fats will result in diabetes, obesity and heart diseases. The DASH diet encourages the consumption of healthier fats such as monounsaturated fats.

Some pointers to be borne in mind, when it comes to the inclusion of fats and oils are as follows:

- Trans fat and saturated fats play an important role in increasing your cholesterol levels. The risk of coronary artery disease is also increased with the consumption of trans fats and saturated fats in large quantities. Hence, the DASH diet restricts the consumption of such fats. Ideally, these fats should form only 6% of the calories you consume in a day. Hence, limit the consumption of butter, meat, cheese, cream, eggs, whole milk, lard, palm oil, coconut oil and solid shortenings.
- Avoid the consumption of baked goods, fried items and crackers, for they are packed with trans fat.

➤ When you buy salad dressings and margarine, make sure you check the label. Pick only those products that are low in terms of saturated fat and free of trans fat.

Sweets:

No. of servings: Up to 5 a week

Yes, the DASH diet permits you to consume sweets. Make sure that you consume limited portions of sweets.

➤ When you consume sweets, make sure you choose those that they are either low fat or fat free. Some examples of such sweets are jelly beans, sorbets, fruit ices, low fat cookies, hard candy or graham crackers.
➤ You can use artificial sweeteners such as sucralose (Splenda) or aspartame (Equal, NutraSweet) instead of sugar. However, make sure that you do not include large quantities of these artificial sweeteners.
➤ Make sure that you do not consume foods that have added sugar in them. These are nothing but empty calories and have absolutely no nutritional value.

How well does the diet conform to accepted dietary guidelines?

Let us look at how well the diet conforms to the laid down dietary guidelines.

Fat: The prescribed recommendation is that only 20% to 35% of the calories that you consume in a day should come from total fat. The DASH diet ensures that you will not exceed this limit. By following this diet, you can also ensure that you do not draw more than the recommended 10 percent of calories from saturated fat.

Protein: The diet is well within the prescribed range, when it comes to the consumption of protein.

Salt: As I mentioned before, the American diet is loaded with salt and exceeds the recommended quantities. The prescribed limit is a maximum of 2,300 mg in a day. If you are already suffering from hypertension, then your daily intake of salt should not exceed 1,500 mg a day. As mentioned earlier, the two variations of the DASH diet will help you meet these requirements.

Fiber: The daily recommended intake of fiber, for adults, is 22 to 34 grams. This is to ensure that your digestive system functions well. The DASH diet most certainly meets this limit because of the inclusion of foodstuffs packed with fiber, such as fruits, vegetables and grains.

Carbohydrates: The diet is well within the prescribed range, when it comes to the consumption of carbohydrates.

Potassium: Potassium is an important nutrient. It works exactly opposite to salt, thereby decreasing the blood pressure levels. It reduces the risk of developing kidney stones and also plays an important role in decreasing bone loss. This is precisely why the recommended intake of this essential nutrient is as high as 4,700 mg a day. Most Americans fail to meet this requirement. However, the DASH diet is all about consuming foods that are packed with potassium. Hence, it is one of those rare diets that will help you meet the required intake of potassium. In fact, it helps you consume as high as 4,900 mg of potassium.

Calcium: Calcium is not just an integral mineral essential for building and maintaining bones, but also to ensure the proper functioning of your muscles and blood vessels. The prescribed intake of calcium should be anywhere between

1,000 mg to 1,300 mg. The typical American diet does not allow you to meet this requirement. However, the DASH diet will help you to consume the requisite intake of calcium very easily.

Vitamin D: Sunlight is the natural source of vitamin D. If you don't get enough sunlight, then your food should contain at least 15 micrograms of vitamin D. This is to ensure that your risks of bone fractures are reduced. DASH diet prescribes the consumption of salmon. The socketeye salmon is particularly rich in this nutrient. Consumption of 3 ounces of this salmon will help you meet the requirement.

Vitamin B-12: Vitamin B-12 is essential for proper cell metabolism. You are required to consume at least 2.4 micrograms of this nutrient. The DASH diet will definitely help you get more than 2.4 micrograms of vitamin B-12.

In short, the daily nutrient goals for the DASH diet are as follows:

- ✓ Total fat – 27% of calories
- ✓ Saturated fat – 6% of calories
- ✓ Protein - 18% of calories
- ✓ Carbohydrates – 55% of calories
- ✓ Sodium – 2,300 mg (1,500 mg for people suffering from hypertension)
- ✓ Potassium – 4,700 mg
- ✓ Magnesium – 500 mg
- ✓ Fiber – 30 g
- ✓ Cholesterol- 150 mg
- ✓ Calcium – 1,250 mg

As you can see, the diet meets all the dietary requirements prescribed by the government.

How easy is the diet to follow?

The only hard part about this diet is giving up the salty and fatty foods, which were your favorites once. Otherwise, this diet is not difficult to follow, for there are lots of foodstuffs involved. In other words, you have an abundant range of healthy foods to choose from, which makes it more interesting.

Another problem that most people face with dieting is that they feel famished soon enough. This is one of the reasons why people find it difficult to follow the diet for a longer period of time. However, this is not the case with the DASH diet. As you know, it is packed with fiber. Hence, you feel full after a meal, despite the reduction in calories. Hence, you will not be tempted to overeat, which in turn is a contributing factor to your weight loss.

Finally, this diet is not a bland option. Though it imposes a restriction in the consumption of salt, it encourages the consumption of spices and herbs in generous quantities. Hence, there is no dearth for flavor, when it comes to the DASH diet.

How does exercise fit in?

Whether you are following the diet to lose weight or to reduce your hypertension, exercise is necessary. Try to allocate at least 30 minutes every day for being physically active. Hitting the gym is not the only way to be physically active. You could resort to brisk walking or gardening or cycling or swimming. Here are a list of common chores and sporting activities that you can resort to, to stay physically active and fit:

A. Common chores:

- ✓ Gardening (30 to 45 minutes)
- ✓ Raking leaves (30 minutes)
- ✓ Shoveling snow (15 minutes)
- ✓ Washing and waxing your car (45 to 60 minutes)
- ✓ Pushing a stroller for at least 1 ½ miles (30 minutes)
- ✓ Washing windows (45 to 60 minutes)
- ✓ Washing floors (45 to 60 minutes)
- ✓ Climbing stairs (15 minutes)

B. Sporting activities:

- ✓ Running 1 ½ miles (15 minutes)
- ✓ Bicycling at least 5 miles (30 minutes)
- ✓ Playing volleyball (45 to 60 minutes)
- ✓ Walking at least 2 miles (30 minutes)
- ✓ Swimming (20 minutes)
- ✓ Playing basketball (15 to 20 minutes)
- ✓ Water aerobics (30 minutes)
- ✓ Playing touch football (45 minutes)
- ✓ Dancing (30 minutes)
- ✓ Jumping rope (15 minutes)

If you are finding it difficult to work out or be physically engaged for a span of 30 minutes, try doing it in installments. Break that 30 minutes into packets of 10 minutes and achieve it through various means. For instance, you can achieve your daily target of 30 minutes by a combination of activities such as climbing stairs, walking inside your office compound for 15 minutes during your coffee break or gardening for 15 minutes. If you increase the time spent on these activities, you will be able to lose more weight in lesser time.

Since the above suggested activities are moderate level physical activities, you don't have to check with your doctor before performing them. However, if you are older than 50 or if heart disease runs in your family or if you are suffering from some other health conditions, you should consult with your doctor first before engaging in such physical activities.

Some action points with respect to exercising are as follows:

- ➢ **Schedule:** Come up with a schedule for your exercise. It could be as straightforward as setting aside 30 minutes for exercising or it could be a combination of exercises spread across the day. Try sticking to the schedule as much as possible.
- ➢ **External support:** Get a friend or family member to join you during your exercise time. This way, you will be motivated to stick to your schedule.
- ➢ **Set goals:** It is important that you set goals for your exercise regime as well. This will motivate you to exercise every day, without any deviations. When you have goals in place, you will also have parameters to track your progress.
- ➢ **Cross train:** Ensure that you try out different exercises every day. This is to ensure that a sole part in the body does not get strained due to excessive exercising.
- ➢ **Reward yourself:** Keep track of your progress. Do not forget to reward yourself when you show some progress. This will help you to follow your schedule with more enthusiasm. Make sure that you don't use food as a reward.

I hope all your preliminary questions about this diet have been answered.

Chapter 2: Principles of DASH Diet

Let us look at the broad principles that govern the DASH diet, in this chapter.

Reduce the sodium content in your diet

As you know, the diet prescribes the limited intake of sodium every day. This can be easily achieved by the following means:

➢ Always go for fresh foods as opposed to processed and refined foods.
➢ Do not add salt to your food at the table.
➢ Be generous when it comes to the inclusion of spices and herbs in your meal.
➢ Keep a tab on the quantity, when you consume canned foods, entrees, vegetables with sauces and frozen foods. If you are going to buy these foods, make sure you read the labels. Pick only the ones that read 'low sodium'. Make sure you rinse the canned foods with clean water before you consume them.
➢ Do not consume large quantities of sausages, bacon, hot dogs, corned beef, bologna, pastrami, salami, ham and processed turkey.
➢ Make sure that you do not consume foods that are pickled, smoked and cured.

Increase foods that are high in magnesium, potassium and fiber

It is important that you increase the consumption of foods rich in nutrients such as potassium and magnesium, for they are capable of regulating your blood pressure levels.

- ➤ Increase the consumption of fresh fruits and vegetables.
- ➤ Make sure you consume citrus fruits at least thrice a week. However, as I mentioned before, people who are under medication, need to check with their doctors before consuming citrus fruits.
- ➤ Include nuts, seeds, peas and dried beans at least four times a week. These are packed with fiber, magnesium and potassium.
- ➤ If you wish to increase your intake of potassium, you may consume bananas, oranges, potatoes and tomatoes. However, if you are suffering from diseases related to the kidney, you need to check with your doctor before you increase the intake of potassium.
- ➤ Inclusion of whole grains and whole grain products in your diet will increase the intake of fiber and magnesium.
- ➤ Do not consume potassium supplements, unless prescribed by the doctor.

Increase the consumption of foods that are rich in calcium

- ➤ To meet your daily requirement of calcium, include low fat or fat free cheeses and yogurts. Ensure that the

dairy products that you choose are devoid of fat or comprises only 1% fat.
- ➢ If you are lactose intolerant, make sure you consume lactose reduced milk or Lactaid.
- ➢ Consume calcium supplements, if you are not going to consume any dairy products.

Drink adequate quantities of fluids

- ➢ Drink at least eight cups of water every day. An easy way to do this is to keep a pitcher full of water at your desk. This will remind you to drink enough water while you are working.
- ➢ Drinks lots of fruit juices. This will not only increase the intake of nutrients and fiber but also keep your body hydrated.

Chapter 3: DASH Diet and health

In this chapter, let us look at how the DASH diet has a positive impact on our health. Here are answers to a bunch of questions about DASH diet's role in improving our health.

Does the DASH diet help in reducing hypertension?

Yes. As I mentioned before, this diet was originally designed to prevent and control hypertension in people. As you already know, the DASH diet achieves this objective in the following manner:

- It regulates the intake of sodium, which is an important factor in determining our blood pressure levels.
- It restricts the consumption of saturated and total fat in large quantities, which in turn can help you regulate your hypertension.
- It encourages the consumption of foods, which are rich in nutrients such as potassium and magnesium and fiber, such as fruits, vegetables. These are capable of reducing the blood pressure levels.

Does the DASH diet help you lose weight?

Unlike the other diets available in the market, the DASH diet is not an exclusive weight loss diet. Nevertheless, it helps you lose weight because of the controlled consumption of calories and reduced intake of fats. Several studies show that the DASH diet indeed does help the dieter lose those extra pounds.

Does it have cardiovascular benefits?

Yes. As we know, hypertension is one of the important reasons behind several heart diseases, stroke and heart failure. So, by controlling hypertension, the risks of these diseases are considerably reduced. The diet has proven to increase the levels of good HDL cholesterol in our blood. It also decreases the bad LDL cholesterol and triglycerides. As you may be aware, high levels of triglycerides are often associated with several heart diseases. To put it in simpler terms, the DASH diet can be rightly referred to as a heart friendly diet.

Does the diet help in dealing with diabetes?

The DASH diet plays an important role not just in preventing diabetes but also controlling it.

Prevention: One of the important risk factors associated with Type 2 diabetes is obesity. As mentioned before, this diet helps you lose those extra pounds. With obesity out of the way, the risk of contracting Type 2 diabetes is decreased. Apart from this, the calorie restrictions imposed by this diet also reduce the risk factors that are associated with metabolic syndrome. Metabolic syndrome, in turn, increases the probability of developing heart diseases and diabetes. Hence, the DASH diet indirectly reduces the risk of contracting diabetes.

Control: A research that was published in 2011 showed that there was a decrease in the blood sugar levels in people suffering from Type 2 diabetes, after following the DASH diet. Hence, the diet is capable of controlling your blood sugar levels, if you are diabetic.

Are there any risks associated with this diet?

No, there are no risks associated with this diet. However, if you are suffering from other health conditions, it is advisable that you check with your doctor first before you follow the diet.

Chapter 4: DASH Diet Chart

As I mentioned before, the DASH diet restricts the intake of calories to 2,000 a day. In this chapter, I have provided a DASH diet chart, which will give you a fair idea about the number of servings, kinds of dishes etc. To put it in simpler terms, you can use this chart to plan your menus.

I. <u>Grains and grain products:</u>
- *No. of servings:* 6-8 a day
- *Serving sizes:*
    a) ½ to 1 cup of dry cereal
    b) 1 slice bread
    c) ½ cup cooked pasta or cereal or rice
- *Examples:* English muffin, bagel, pita bread, oatmeal, grits, cereals and whole wheat bread.
- *Importance:* They are major sources of fiber and energy.

II. <u>Vegetables:</u>
- *No. of servings:* 4- 5 a day
- *Serving sizes:*
    a) 1 cup raw leafy vegetable
    b) 6 ounces vegetable juice
    c) ½ cup cooked vegetable
- *Examples:* Potatoes, tomatoes, peas, squash, carrots, broccoli, kale, spinach, collards, turnips, sweet potatoes, beans, artichokes.
- *Importance:* They are packed with potassium, magnesium and fiber.

III.   **Fruits:**
- *No. of servings:* 4- 5 a day
- *Serving sizes:*
    a) 1 medium fruit
    b) ½ cup fruit juice
    c) ½ cup fresh, canned or frozen fruit
    d) ¼ cup dried fruit
- *Examples:* Bananas, apricots, dates, oranges, grapes, orange juice, grapefruit, melons, grapefruit juice, mangoes, pineapples, peaches, tangerines, raisins, prunes, strawberries.
- *Importance:* They are packed with potassium, magnesium and fiber.

IV.   **Dairy products (Low fat or fat free):**
- *No. of servings:* 2-3 a day
- *Serving sizes:*
    a) 1 cup milk
    b) 1 ½ ounce cheese
    c) 1 cup yogurt
- *Examples:* Non fat or low fat yogurt, non fat cheese, skim or 1% milk, low fat or skim buttermilk, partly skimmed mozzarella cheese.
- *Importance:* They are rich in calcium and protein.

V. **Poultry, meat and fish:**
- *No. of servings:* Up to 6 a day
- *Serving sizes:*
    a) 1 ounce cooked poultry or meat or fish.
    b) 2 egg whites or 1 egg

- *Examples:* Poultry (with skin removed), egg yolk (up to 4 in a week), lean meats (fat trimmed), broiled or baked or roasted meat.
- *Importance:* They are rich in protein and magnesium.

VI. <u>Legumes, nuts and seeds:</u>
- *No. of servings:* 4- 5 per week
- *Serving sizes:*
    a) 2 tablespoons natural nut butter
    b) 1 ½ ounces or 1/3 cup of nuts
    c) ½ ounce or 2 tablespoons seeds
    d) ½ cup cooked legumes
- *Examples:* Filberts, peanuts, almonds, walnuts, sunflower seeds, mixed nuts, lentils, kidney beans, peas.
- *Importance:* They are rich in potassium, fiber and protein. They are also rich sources of energy.

VII. <u>Fats and oils:</u>
- *No. of servings:* 2- 3 a day
- *Serving sizes:*
    a) 1 tablespoon low fat margarine or mayonnaise
    b) 1 tablespoon vegetable oil or regular mayonnaise or soft margarine
    c) 2 tablespoons light salad dressing
- *Examples:* Low fat mayonnaise, light salad dressing, olive oil, corn oil, safflower oil, canola oil, soft margarine

- *Importance:* They are essential in the absorption of vitamins by the body.

VIII. <u>Sweets:</u>
- *No. of servings:* 5 per week
- *Serving sizes:*
  a) 8 ounces lemonade
  b) ½ ounce jelly beans
  c) 1 tablespoon sugar
  d) 1 tablespoon jam or jelly
- *Examples:* Jelly beans, hard candy, maple syrup, sorbet, sugar, jelly, ices, fruit flavored gelatin, jam, fruit punch.
- *Importance:* Make sure that you pick sweets that are low in terms of fat. People with diabetes are advised to reduce the servings to less than 5 a week, as advised by their doctor.

I hope this diet chart helped you gain some perspective about this diet. As you may have seen, the DASH diet is all about including healthy foodstuffs that not only reduce your blood pressure but also play an important role in you leading a healthy lifestyle. Even though it is not a diet that is built for weight loss, it invariably helps you lose those extra pounds because of the restriction in the intake of calories, saturated fats, processed and refined foods.

Sodium levels:

Now that you have had the chance to look at the sample diet chart, let us look at the sodium content present in the different foodstuffs. This will help you appreciate the aforesaid diet chart better, for you can see how it includes more of foods that are low in sodium content, thereby ensuring that your intake of sodium does not exceed 2,300 mg or 1,500 mg, as the case maybe.

S.NO	FOOD GROUPS	SODIUM CONTENT (MG)
A.	**Fruits**	
(i)	½ cup of fresh or frozen or canned fruit	0 to 5
B.	**Vegetables**	
(i)	½ cup of frozen or canned vegetables with sauce	140 to 460
(ii)	½ cup of fresh or frozen vegetables, cooked without salt	1 to 70
(iii)	½ cup canned tomato juice	330
C.	**Whole and other grains and grain products**	
(i)	1 slice bread	110 to 175
(ii)	1 cup ready to eat cereal	0 to 360
(iii)	½ cup cooked rice, pasta, rice (unsalted)	0 to 5
D.	**Nuts, seeds and legumes**	
(i)	1/3 cup salted peanuts	120
(ii)	1/3 cup unsalted peanuts	0 to 5
(iii)	½ cup canned beans	400
(iv)	½ cup cooked beans (without salt)	0 to 5
E.	Dairy products (low fat or fat free)	
(i)	1 cup milk	107

(ii)	1 ½ ounces cheeses	110 to 450
(iii)	1 cup yogurt	175
(iv)	2 ounces processed cheese	600
F.	Lean meats, fish and poultry	
(i)	3 ounces of canned tuna, water pack (without salt)	35 to 45
(ii)	3 ounces of canned tuna, water pack	230 to 350
(iii)	3 ounces of fish or fresh meat or poultry	30 to 90
(iv)	3 ounces of lean and roasted ham	1,020

It is evident from the above table that the DASH diet restricts the consumption of foodstuffs that are high in sodium content.

Chapter 5: DASH Diet Tips

If you are trying the diet for the first time, I am sure you will be anxious about how to go about it. To put you out of your misery, I have compiled several tips, with respect to the DASH diet, in this chapter. By the end of this chapter, I am sure you will feel more confident than before about following this diet.

Getting Started

In this section of this chapter, you will find those tips that will help you get started with this diet.

> ➤ **Take it slow:** Ensure that the change is gradual. As of now, if you are eating only one or two servings of fruits and vegetables every day, try including one more serving at lunch or dinner. You can increase it to the requisite servings gradually. Similarly, if you are not used to consuming whole grains, don't try to switch over immediately. Start including whole grains in one or two servings. This will help you avoid bloating and diarrhea, which are commonly associated with the sudden consumption of fiber in large quantities. In order to avoid gas, which is commonly associated with the intake of beans and vegetables, you may also try over the counter products.

> ➤ **Make sure you reward successes:** Since this is the first time you will be trying this diet plan, make sure that you have a proper reward system in place. It will not be possible for you to adhere to the diet 100% in the very first week. Make room for these little

failures. If you are prepared for these little failures, you will not be discouraged to follow the diet because of a small slip up. On the contrary, if you strive to achieve perfection from the beginning, you will only be disappointed. Disappointment can often discourage you from following a diet plan. When you see that you have deviated from the diet, try to identify the reason behind the slip up. Your job does not end with just identifying the reason. Try to figure out ways to ensure that the slip up does not happen again. Resume the DASH diet where you left it.

On the other hand, it is necessary that you acknowledge your little successes and reward it wisely. Make sure that the rewards are non food items. It can be as simple as renting a movie or visiting a friend. When you learn to acknowledge these little successes, you will be motivated to follow the diet.

➢ **Physical exercise:** The DASH diet, coupled with physical exercise, cannot only help you lower your blood pressure but also help you lose weight easily. Hence, ensure that you spend some time for exercising every day.

➢ **Get external advice:** If you are finding it difficult to stick to the diet, do not hesitate to get in touch with a dietician or doctor. They may help you overcome the difficulties you are facing with respect to the diet.

➢ **Form a support system:** The success of any diet plan depends on your levels of motivation. If you are not motivated, you will not be able to get through the diet at all. As I mentioned before, the DASH diet is a long term approach. Hence, it is important that your motivation levels are high, if you wish to adopt the DASH diet in the long run. Seek the help of family and friends to meet your diet goals. Keep them briefed about your diet goals and the reason why you want to follow this diet. This way, your friends and family will be in a position to motivate you, when you find it difficult to follow the diet. Also, when you keep them in the loop, the chances of them tempting you into deviating from the diet are very less.

➢ **Maintain a journal:** Write down everything you eat. This way, you will find it easier to identify the pain points in your diet. For instance, if you are facing bloating issues, it could be because of the sudden inclusion of fibers in your diet. When you look at your journal, you will be able to monitor your intake of fiber in such a fashion that you don't face bloating issues. Another advantage of maintaining a journal is that you will be able to find out if you are allergic to certain kinds of foods.

Another reason why having a diet journal is advantageous is because it will help you shop wisely next time. Now that you have a clear idea of how much you eat, what foods you are allergic to, you will be able to pick out the ingredients for your meals in a prudent fashion.

➢ **Cook your own meals:** The best way to ensure that you stick to the diet is by cooking your own meals. When you cook your own meals, you will be able to ensure that all the ingredients that you use and the techniques that you adopt are DASH friendly. If it is possible to make all of your ingredients from scratch, then go for it. For instance, if you are cooking pasta, try to make your own pasta instead of going for store made pasta. Similarly, make your own sauce instead of opting for readymade sauce.

Tips for shopping

In this section, you will find various tips that will help you shop wisely for preparing your DASH diet recipes. Let us look at them now:

> **Make a list:** Plan your meals well ahead. Before you head out for shopping, you should have a clear idea about the dishes you are going to cook over the week. Only if you are clear about the dishes that you are going to cook will you be able to prepare a list of the ingredients that are required. Ensure that you put down every single ingredient in your list. Remember that you will require ingredients for preparing DASH snacks and breakfasts too. So, do not forget to include them in your list. When you have a list in hand, you will be able to shop better in a focused fashion. Most often, people tend to stray away from the diet and end up shopping processed foods and snacks, mainly because they don't have a proper grocery list on hand. Hence, it all rides on how detailed your grocery list is.

> **Eat before you go shopping:** You may wonder how this is a relevant tip. Think about the number of times you have grabbed a snack from the shelves because you were hungry while shopping. This could be an important reason behind you deviating from the diet. When we are hungry, we don't bother checking labels and ingredients. We just grab the snack within our reach to satisfy our hunger. Hence, make sure that

you eat well before you go shopping. This way, you will buy only the things mentioned in your grocery list and not consume anything that could possibly make you deviate from your diet.

➤ **Buy Fresh:** As you know, the DASH diet discourages the consumption of processed and refined foods because of their sodium and fat content. Hence, the key is to buy fresh ingredients. Fresh foods contain low quantities of sodium, fat and are devoid of added sugar, salt and preservatives. They also have more flavors as opposed to processed foods. Another important reason why fresh foods are better is because they are packed with fiber, vitamins and minerals. If you are opting for the canned versions of fresh foods, such as canned vegetables, make sure that you pick only those that have reduced fat and sodium.

➤ **Shop the perimeter:** Though most of the DASH friendly ingredients are stacked in the center aisles, make sure you walk around a bit. This is because you will not find fresh produce or low fat dairy products or lean meats in the center aisles. Hence, make it a point to buy everything mentioned in your shopping list, which will require you to focus on all the sections of the grocery store and not just the center aisles.

➤ **Read labels:** As you may be aware, it is a prerequisite for most packaged foods to display their nutrition facts in their labels. Reading the labels will help you pick only those ingredients that are DASH friendly. In other words, you can easily avoid packaged foods that have added sugar/salt/preservatives, high quantities of sodium and fat and more calories. Even among DASH friendly foods, read the labels and compare the nutrition facts and pick only those that are lower in fat and sodium and has lesser calories.

Tips for the kitchen

Now that we have seen tips related to shopping, let us look at some of the tips associated with your kitchen and cookware.

- ➤ **Stock your pantry well:** A well stocked pantry is instrumental in making you follow the diet without deviations. When you don't have a pantry that is not stocked well, you will not be motivated to cook. You would rather be motivated to order in food. As you know, fast foods are unhealthy and do not meet the requirements of this diet. Hence, make sure that you stock your pantry well with fruits, vegetables, grains, legumes, seeds, poultry, nuts, meats, fish and low fat dairy products. Make sure you have generous quantities of seasonings and condiments in your pantry.
- ➤ **Choose the right cookware:** Make sure that you have the appropriate cookware and gadgets in place. This will help you prepare your DASH diet recipes with ease. Some of the cookware that need to find a place in your kitchen are as follows:
  - *Nonstick cookware:* When you use nonstick cookware, you will end up using less oil or butter while cooking your meat or vegetables.
  - *Garlic press or spice mill:* Most of us tend to add salt at the table, to add more flavors to our food. These items will help you add more flavors to your food. Hence, this will discourage you from adding salt to your food at the table.

- *Vegetable steamer insert:* When you have a vegetable steamer insert, which you can fit into the bottom of a saucepan, you will find it easier to prepare steamed vegetables, without adding oil or butter to the pan.

Cooking tips

In this section of this chapter, you will find several tips pertaining to cooking. These tips will help you reduce the sodium and fat content in your meals.

- ➤ **Rinse it off:** If you are using canned foods such as vegetables, beans, tuna etc, make sure you rinse the food well with water, before cooking it. This will help you wash off any excess salt present in these foods.
- ➤ **Add more spices:** You can easily increase the flavor of your food by adding more spices instead of using salt or fat. You can add herbs, flavored vinegars, onions, spices, ginger, garlic powder, fresh pepper, garlic, limes, bouillon (sodium free) to your meal to increase the flavor of it. You can also add soy sauce to your meal, provided it has low sodium content.
- ➤ **Be careful with your broth:** Even though the label of your broth may state "low sodium", it will still have lots of sodium. Hence, if you are using broth for your dish, make sure that you include as little as possible.
- ➤ **Cut back on meat:** Reduce your intake of meat. Prepare casseroles and stews with only two thirds of the meat prescribed in the recipe. You can make do for the lack of meat by adding more vegetables, tofu, brown rice, whole wheat pasta or bulgur.

- ➢ **Use lower fat substitutes:** This is necessary when it comes to choosing your dairy products. Go for only low fat versions instead of the high fat ones.
- ➢ **Smoothies:** When you prepare smoothies, make sure you use only fresh fruits and skim milk. Do not add any sugar to your smoothie.

Tips for dining out

In this section of the chapter, you will find tips relevant to help you follow the diet even while dining out.

Reduce your salt intake

- ➢ While ordering your food, mention that you want them to prepare it without added MSG or salt or other ingredients that have added salt in them. Since most restaurants will cook based on the needs of the customer, you will not find it difficult to stick to your diet, even while dining out.
- ➢ When you go over the menu card, don't just watch out for the ingredients. Watch out for the cooking techniques as well. For example, cured foods do not meet the requirements of the DASH diet. Hence, do not order foods that are cured or smoked or pickled. Do not pick dishes that contain broth and soy sauce as well, for they will contain large amounts of sodium.
- ➢ Refrain from touching the saltshaker present in your table.
- ➢ Restrict the consumption of condiments that have salt in large amounts, such as pickles, sauces, ketchup and mustard.
- ➢ Do not choose appetizers that are salty. Instead, go for fruits and vegetables.

Reduce the intake of unhealthy fats

> ➤ While ordering your food, make sure that you tell them to prepare it using olive oil instead of butter or other unhealthy fats.
> ➤ When you order salads, ask them to use vinegar and oil as dressing, instead of using salad dressings. If the same is not possible, request for the salad dressing as a side, instead of incorporating it as part of the salad.
> ➤ Even very lean meats contain fats. Hence, make sure you consume only limited servings of meat dishes. Ensure that the fat and the skin are trimmed off your dish.
> ➤ When you order steamed vegetables or fruits, ensure that butter or sauces do not accompany them.
> ➤ As I mentioned before, look out for cooking techniques as well, before you order your food. Order dishes that are steamed or grilled or baked or broiled or roasted or poached or stir fried instead of those dishes that are deep fried.
> ➤ When you order broiled or steamed fish, make sure you request for fresh herbs, lemon and seasonings.

Pay equal attention to all courses

It is important that you ensure that all the courses are DASH friendly. Here are a few pointers for you to help you achieve this feat.

> ➤ Go for appetizers, which feature fruits or fresh vegetables or fish as the hero.
> ➤ When you want beverages to wash down your meal, go for diet soda, water, club soda, tea, and coffee and fruit juice. If you are choosing an alcoholic beverage, consume only moderate quantities of it. The

prescribed quantity is one drink a day for women and two drinks a day for men. The following portions count as one drink:

- 5 ounces of wine (100 calories) (or)
- 12 ounces of beer, regular or light (150 calories) (or)
- 1 ½ ounces of 80 proof whiskey (100 calories)

➢ When you order salads, go for a fruit salad or spinach or tossed greens. Ensure that the salad does not contain eggs, meats or cheese. As I mentioned before, order for the dressing to be served as a side.

➢ Try to skip the bread course, if possible. If it is not possible, order breadsticks, rolls or bread that is made from whole grains.

➢ When you are choosing your dessert, go for sorbet, fresh fruit, fruit ice, sherbet, plain cake with fruit puree or meringues.

Avoid oversized portions

Since the DASH diet prescribes serving sizes, it is necessary that you keep an eye on the size of the portions you consume. This is particularly necessary when you are eating out, because restaurants tend to serve more than what is required. Here are a few pointers to ensure that you don't overeat:

➢ Even if you have gone to the restaurant for dinner, order only for a lunch portion of the dish.

➢ Do not go for an entrée. Instead, go for an appetizer.

➢ Try to go to the restaurant with a companion and share your meal with them. This way, you will not eat more than what is required.

> If you are going to the restaurant alone, place half the meal in a takeout container, before you begin eating. This is another way to ensure that you eat only what is required.

Be prudent with fast food

It is entirely possible for you to deviate from the DASH diet, if you consume fast foods without exercising enough caution. You don't have to completely shun fast foods. You can still go ahead and have a fast food meal, once in a while, if you stick to the following tips:

> When you order, ensure that you mention that your dish does not have added salt.
> Before you pick your restaurant, ensure that you do a bit of research. These days, details about most restaurants are published online. So, check out the nutrition information about the various fast food outlets and choose the healthier one.
> When you order for your meal, go for regular size or children's size. This will ensure that you don't gobble up too much of junk food.
> Refrain from ordering salads at these fast food outlets. This is because most of these salads have cheese or salad dressings in them, which are unhealthy in nature.
> Do not go for dishes that are battered or fried. Pick only those dishes that are steamed or broiled or grilled.
> When you are picking sides for your dishes, go for healthier options like fresh fruits or baked potato.

Social gatherings

It is not entirely possible to avoid social gatherings just because you are dieting. You may be required to participate in social gatherings. Here are a few pointers to deal with these events and still staying on the track:

> Before you step out for the event, ensure that you eat at home. This way, you will not feel hungry when you go to the event. You may just grab a fruit juice or a healthy appetizer.

> If you are not able to eat before you go out, ensure that you walk around and choose only those foods that are DASH friendly. Keep a tab on the portions that you are consuming. As you know, the DASH diet is all about planning your meals in such a way that it does not exceed the calorie requirements for the day.

Time Saving tips

In this section, I have compiled several tips that will help you save time, when it comes to following the DASH diet. I am sure that time is a constraint for most of us in today's world. Hence, I am sure that you will appreciate the following tips:

> To considerably save your cooking time as well as your efforts, you may use various kitchen appliances. For example, if you use the slow cooker, your cooking efforts can be considerably reduced. All that you need to do is to toss the ingredients into the slow cooker and let it do the cooking. Some other appliances that you may use include pressure cooker, rice cooker, food processor, slow cooker or a blender.

> Ensure that you wash the vegetables well and prepare them, as soon as you return from the grocery store.

This way, you will need less than few minutes to actually cook your dish.

➢ Make sure that your kitchen scissors are kept handy. This will help you prepare the other ingredients required for your meal.

➢ To save the time spent on cleaning vegetables, you may opt for ready to eat vegetables. Also buy lettuce that is pre-washed. Since lettuce takes time to wash and clean thoroughly, this could help you save some time.

➢ If your recipe calls for grated cheese, buy readymade grated cheese. Ensure that the readymade cheese is low in fat content.

➢ When you are cooking, make sure that you cook enough for two meals at least. This way, you can considerably save the time spent on cooking the next meal.

➢ When you are preparing lean proteins or beans for your meal, make sure that you cook extra. These can be used for the recipes throughout the week.

➢ Ensure that you have a decent stock of pasta, rice and other grains. Store them in the refrigerator and use them in soups, casseroles or salads.

➢ When you are cooking something in the oven, make sure that you bake the potatoes or sweet potatoes required for the next meal. All you need to do is to wrap them inside an aluminum foil and keep it inside the oven.

➢ When you are sautéing or blanching vegetables for dinner, make sure that you prepare some more vegetables. These can be used for preparing the next day's lunch.

- When you are preparing cabbage for a meal, make sure that you cut the entire head, even if it is more than what you require for the dish. Store the remaining cabbage in a zip lock bag and store it in the freezer. You can use it for future recipes.
- When you are preparing green salad, make sure that you prepare it without any dressing. Prepare generous amounts of the salad and store it in an airtight container and refrigerate.
- Do not discard leftovers. Pack the leftovers from dinner in a microwave friendly container for lunch. You can heat it and have it as lunch.
- If there's leftover chili from dinner, do not throw it away. Stuff it into a baked potato or wrap it inside a warm tortilla and have it for lunch or breakfast.
- If you are out of time, you may buy from the nearby deli, a rotisserie chicken. Turn it into a complete meal by serving it along with couscous (made from whole wheat) and fresh vegetables.
- You could go for readymade ingredients such as pre-cut or frozen vegetables, grated parmesan cheese, cooked pasta or marinara sauce (low in sodium content), if you don't have this time to prepare these ingredients from scratch.
- If you opt for the grain mixes or boxed rice, then use only half the contents of the seasoning packet that comes along with the pack. This is because the seasonings will be loaded with salt. Serve it with a generous portion of vegetables and lean proteins.
- If you are going for a pizza, order it with half the cheese and twice the quantity of vegetables, along with a green salad.

Tips to get back on track

If you are someone who has never felt the need to eat healthy, until now, the chances of you deviating from the diet are pretty high. This is not because you lack the resolve. Eating healthy is a relatively new habit for you and it would take time for you to adjust. So, should you ever deviate, here are a few pointers to help you get back on track.

Look for the reason

As I mentioned before, it is important that you identify the reason for such a deviation. Was it because you had gone out for a social event? Or were you stressed and you took to binge eating? Was it because you ran out of DASH friendly ingredients? Whatever be the reason, it is important that you identify it. Only then, will you be able to figure out a way to prevent such deviations in the future. For instance, if the reason for you getting off the track is the lack of support from your family, you could sit and have a chat with them about the importance of this diet and the necessity for you to follow it, without any deviations.

Don't fret too much

If you have slipped once, do not ascertain too much meaning to it. Do not blame yourself or take it too hard. As you know already, the DASH diet is a long term approach. It is only natural that there are a few slip ups in the first few weeks. As I mentioned before, try figuring out the reason for such a slip up, instead of worrying too much about it.

Don't try to push yourself too much

As I mentioned before, take it slow. The DASH diet is most certainly a drastic change in your lifestyle. Hence, do not try to push yourself too much or try too hard. Change gradually and you will find yourself getting accustomed to this healthy lifestyle in no time.

Break it into small steps

Goal setting is essential for you to have focus. You need to have goals for your diet as well. Only then, will you be able to stick to it. Break your major goals into micro ones. For instance, if the reason behind you following the diet is to lose 10 pounds, try setting goals for every week, which will enable you to lose 2 to 3 pounds. Similarly, if you are adopting the diet to reduce your blood pressure, ensure that your weekly goal is to maintain your blood pressure at a certain level. These micro goals will help you stick to the diet.

Sample grocery list

Here is a sample grocery list that will come handy when you are planning your meals.

Vegetables:

- ✓ Asparagus
- ✓ Artichokes
- ✓ Bell peppers
- ✓ Beets
- ✓ Broccoli
- ✓ Cabbage
- ✓ Brussels sprouts
- ✓ Cauliflower

- ✓ Carrots
- ✓ Celery
- ✓ Cucumbers
- ✓ Corn
- ✓ Green beans
- ✓ Eggplant
- ✓ Mushrooms
- ✓ Jicama
- ✓ Collards
- ✓ Swiss chard
- ✓ Kale
- ✓ Turnip greens
- ✓ Lettuce
- ✓ Leeks
- ✓ Green peas
- ✓ Red onions
- ✓ White onions
- ✓ Yellow onions
- ✓ Snow peas
- ✓ Snap peas
- ✓ Green onions
- ✓ Sweet potatoes
- ✓ Potatoes
- ✓ Parsnips
- ✓ Radishes
- ✓ Rutabaga
- ✓ Zucchini
- ✓ Spinach
- ✓ Acorn
- ✓ Spaghetti squash
- ✓ Pumpkin
- ✓ Butternut squash
- ✓ Tomatoes

Fruits

- ✓ Bananas
- ✓ Apricots
- ✓ Strawberries
- ✓ Apples
- ✓ Blackberries
- ✓ Blueberries
- ✓ Raspberries
- ✓ Figs
- ✓ Dates
- ✓ Cherries
- ✓ Grapes
- ✓ Oranges
- ✓ Grapefruits
- ✓ Tangerines
- ✓ Lemons
- ✓ Papaya
- ✓ Kiwi fruit
- ✓ Mango
- ✓ Cantaloupe
- ✓ Watermelon
- ✓ Pears
- ✓ Nectarines
- ✓ Pineapple
- ✓ Peaches
- ✓ Honeydew
- ✓ Raisins
- ✓ Prunes
- ✓ Plums
- ✓

Breads (Whole grain/Whole wheat)

- ✓ English muffins
- ✓ Bread
- ✓ Bagels
- ✓ Pita
- ✓ Tortillas (corn or whole-wheat)
- ✓ Pizza crust

Cereal

- ✓ Low fat granola
- ✓ Bran cereal
- ✓ Muesli
- ✓ Old fashioned oats or steel cut
- ✓ Whole grain cereal

Grains

- ✓ Brown rice
- ✓ Couscous (whole wheat)
- ✓ Bulgur
- ✓ Barley
- ✓ Kasha (buckwheat)
- ✓ Spelt
- ✓ Triticale
- ✓ Pasta (whole wheat)
- ✓ Kamut
- ✓ Wild rice
- ✓ Millet
- ✓ Amaranth
- ✓ Quinoa

Meat, Poultry, Seafood, Soy

- ✓ Beef
- ✓ Eggs
- ✓ Chicken
- ✓ Turkey
- ✓ Fish fillets
- ✓ Shrimps
- ✓ Salmon
- ✓ Tempeh
- ✓ Tofu
- ✓ Pork tenderloin

Frozen Foods

- ✓ 100% fruit juice
- ✓ French toast (whole grain)
- ✓ Vegetables
- ✓ Whole grain waffles
- ✓ Pancakes (whole grain)
- ✓ Fish fillets
- ✓ Shellfish
- ✓ Chicken breast (skinless)
- ✓ 100% fruit juice bars
- ✓ Veggie burgers

Dairy

- ✓ Low fat cottage cheese
- ✓ Trans fat free margarine
- ✓ Fat free or low fat yogurt
- ✓ Fat free or low fat flavored milk
- ✓ Blue cheese
- ✓ Goat cheese
- ✓ Feta cheese

- ✓ Cheddar cheese (reduced fat)
- ✓ Parmesan
- ✓ Monterey jack
- ✓ Kefir
- ✓ Partly skimmed mozzarella
- ✓ Low fat sour cream
- ✓ Fat free or low fat milk
- ✓ Low fat buttermilk

Packaged Snacks

- ✓ Pretzels (whole grain)
- ✓ Dried fruit
- ✓ Popcorn
- ✓ Crackers (whole grain)

Nuts & Seeds

- ✓ Cashews
- ✓ Walnuts
- ✓ Soy nuts
- ✓ Hazelnuts
- ✓ Almonds
- ✓ Pecans
- ✓ Peanuts
- ✓ Peanut butter
- ✓ Almond butter
- ✓ Sunflower seeds
- ✓ Pumpkin seeds

Canned Goods

- ✓ Tomato paste
- ✓ Unsweetened applesauce
- ✓ Low sodium or reduced sodium broth

- ✓ Canned salmon
- ✓ Canned tuna
- ✓ Low sodium or reduced sodium soup
- ✓ Diced chilies
- ✓ Low sodium or reduced sodium tomatoes
- ✓ Low sodium or reduced sodium tomato sauce
- ✓ Kidney beans
- ✓ Pinto beans
- ✓ Black beans
- ✓ Split peas
- ✓ Garbanzo beans

Condiments, Sauces, Spreads

- ✓ Low fat mayonnaise
- ✓ Pesto
- ✓ Mustard
- ✓ Bean dip
- ✓ Hot sauce or chili sauce
- ✓ Low sugar or fruit only spreads
- ✓ Olive oil
- ✓ Canola oil
- ✓ Sesame oil
- ✓ Fresh salsa
- ✓ Hummus
- ✓ Reduced sodium marinara sauce
- ✓ Low fat salad dressing
- ✓ Reduced sodium soy sauce
- ✓ Balsamic vinegar
- ✓ Sun dried tomatoes
- ✓ Rice wine vinegar
- ✓ Red wine vinegar
- ✓ Cider vinegar

Herbs and spices

- ✓ Cayenne pepper
- ✓ Allspice
- ✓ Bay leaf
- ✓ Chives
- ✓ Basil
- ✓ Chili powder
- ✓ Chili flakes
- ✓ Cinnamon
- ✓ Cilantro
- ✓ Cloves
- ✓ Coriander
- ✓ Curry powder
- ✓ Garlic
- ✓ Dill
- ✓ Cumin
- ✓ Ginger
- ✓ Mustard
- ✓ Nutmeg
- ✓ Mint
- ✓ Oregano
- ✓ Parsley
- ✓ White pepper
- ✓ Black pepper
- ✓ Paprika
- ✓ Sage
- ✓ Rosemary
- ✓ Tarragon
- ✓ Sesame seeds
- ✓ Thyme

Beverages

- ✓ Herbal tea
- ✓ Low sodium vegetable juice
- ✓ Sparkling water

I hope the tips mentioned in this chapter will be useful in helping you stick to this diet.

Chapter 6: Dash Diet Breakfast Recipes

The DASH diet has proven to lower blood pressure as well as lower the reliance people have on medications. It does so by recommending that you cut back on the carbs and increase your intake of healthy fats and proteins. By focusing on eating beans, seeds, low fat and nonfat dairy then combining this with vegetables and fruits, you will experience weight loss that is sustainable and successful. The diet also focuses on maintenance of your muscles, so that metabolism does not slow down. The recipes in this book will be your guide to healthy living. This section of the book includes recipes suitable to give you energy for the morning.

Apple Spice Baked Oatmeal (160 calories per serving)

Yields: 9 servings

Ingredients:

- 1 teaspoon cinnamon
- ¼ teaspoon salt
- 1 teaspoon baking powder
- 2 cups rolled oats
- 1 apple, chopped (about 1 ½ cups)
- 2 tablespoons oil
- 1 teaspoon vanilla
- 1½ cups non- fat milk
- ½ cup applesauce, sweetened

- 1 egg, beaten

Topping:

- 2 tablespoons chopped nuts
- 2 tablespoons brown sugar

Instructions

Preheat the oven to 375 degrees. Spray an 8 by 8 inch baking pan with oil. Put the milk, vanilla, applesauce, the egg and apple in one bowl and mix them.

Combine baking powder, rolled oats, salt and cinnamon in a separate bowl and mix them together. Add the liquid ingredients and mix the combination properly. Pour the mixture into the baking dish and bake for 25 minutes.

Remove it from the oven and sprinkle with the nuts and the brown sugar. Return it in the oven and bake for an additional 4 minutes, under supervision, until the sugar bubbles and the top turns brown.

Cut into 9 and serve warm.

Banana nut pancake (146 calories per serving)

Yields: 6 servings

Ingredients

- 2 tablespoons chopped walnuts
- 1 teaspoon vanilla
- 2 teaspoons oil
- 3 large egg whites
- 1 cup low fat milk
- 1 large banana, mashed
- ¼ teaspoon cinnamon
- ¼ teaspoon salt
- 2 teaspoons baking powder
- 1 cup whole wheat flour

Instructions

Put all dry ingredients in a bowl. In a separate bowl, add milk, mashed bananas, oil, vanilla and egg whites and mix them together. Combine wet ingredients with dry ingredients and mix well with a spoon.

Heat your pan over medium heat then spray it lightly with oil. Pour ¼ cup of pancake batter into it for each pancake and wait until the batter starts to bubble and the edges turn brown before you turn it over. Do the same with the remaining batter.

Serve while warm.

Applesauce French Toast (150 calories per serving)

Yields: 6 servings

Ingredients

- 6 slices whole wheat bread
- ¼ cup unsweetened applesauce
- 2 tablespoons white sugar
- 1 teaspoon ground cinnamon
- ½ cup milk
- 2 eggs

Instructions

Combine cinnamon, milk, eggs, applesauce and sugar in a mixing bowl and mix them thoroughly. Soak one slice of bread at a time in the mixture until the bread has absorbed the mixture.

Grease your skillet lightly and cook the batter on medium heat until golden brown. Do the same for the other side.

Serve hot.

Oat Blueberry Pancakes (160 calories per serving)

Yields: 10 servings

Ingredients

- 1 cup frozen blueberries
- 1 egg
- 1 cup whole wheat flour
- ½ teaspoon baking soda
- ½ cup steel cut oats
- ½ cup Greek vanilla yogurt
- 1 ½ cups water
- 1/8 teaspoon sea salt
- ½ cup +2 tablespoons agave nectar
- 1 cup milk
- ½ teaspoon baking powder

Instructions

Boil water in a medium pot and then add some salt and steel cut oats. Cook the oats on a low simmer until they are tender then set the pot aside.

Combine whole wheat pastry flour and baking powder, yogurt, milk and egg in a medium mixing bowl. Mix thoroughly to form a batter. Into this, fold the berries and the cooked oats carefully.

Spray your skillet with cooking spray and heat it over medium heat. On its surface, put ¼ cup batter onto the surface and cook until the pancakes are slightly golden. Do the same for the other side. Garnish your pancakes with 1 tablespoon agave nectar then serve.

Mushroom, cheese, and spinach scramble
(150 calories per serving)

Yields: 1 serving

Ingredients

- 2 tablespoons feta cheese
- Cooking spray
- 1 cup fresh spinach, chopped
- 2 egg whites
- Pepper to taste
- 1 whole egg
- ½ cup fresh mushrooms, sliced

Instructions

Spray a sauté pan with cooking spray and heat over medium heat. Add spinach and mushroom and sauté for about 3 minutes.

In a mixing bowl whisk the egg whites and egg with pepper and feta cheese. Pour the mixture over the vegetables. Cook the eggs while stirring for about 4 minutes.

Serve hot.

Bread pudding (250 calories per serving)

Yields: 4 servings

Ingredients

- 2 tablespoons brown sugar
- ½ cup apple, peeled and diced
- 2 teaspoons powdered sugar
- ¼ cup raisins
- 3 cups cubed whole wheat bread, 4 slices
- ½ teaspoon vanilla extract
- 1/8 teaspoon salt
- 1½ cups low fat milk
- 4 eggs
- ½ teaspoon ground cinnamon

Instructions

Preheat the oven to 350 degrees. Combine eggs, brown sugar, cinnamon, vanilla, salt and milk and mix them thoroughly in a large mixing bowl.

Add diced apples and bread cubes then whisk all the ingredients and ensure they are well combined and that the bread has soaked up.

Coat an 8 by 8 inch baking dish with butter and transfer the mixture into it. Cover with foil and bake for 40 minutes in the oven. Remove the cover and continue baking until it turns to golden brown.

Remove it from the oven, dust with sugar and serve after 10 minutes.

Grain and Fruit Breakfast Salad (187 calories per serving)

Yields: 6 servings

Ingredients

- 1 orange, peeled and cut into sections
- 1 Granny Smith apple
- 3 cups water
- 1 cup raisins
- ¼ teaspoon salt
- 1 container (8 oz.) low fat vanilla yogurt
- ¾ cup bulgur
- 1 red apple, cored and chopped
- ¾ cup quick cooking brown rice

Instructions

Boil salted water in a large pot over high temperatures. Reduce the heat to low and add bulgur and rice. Cook for 10 minutes. Remove from the heat and set aside.

On a baking sheet, place the hot grains to cool. Transfer the chilled grains into a mixing bowl and combine with the fruits. Finally, add the yogurt into mixing bowl and stir until coated.

Mushroom Frittata (160 calories per serving)

Yields: 4 servings

Ingredients

- ¼ cup fresh parmesan cheese, grated
- 1 tablespoon milk
- 5 large egg whites
- 3 eggs
- Black pepper to taste
- 1 teaspoon dried thyme
- 2 teaspoons fresh parsley, chopped
- ½ pounds mushroom, finely chopped
- 4 shallots, finely chopped
- 1 tablespoon unsalted butter

Instructions

Preheat the oven to 350 degrees. Use a large ovenproof skillet to heat butter over medium heat. Add in shallots and stir until golden brown.

Whisk egg whites, eggs, milk and parmesan in a medium bowl. Add the egg mixture to the skillet with the eggs covering the mushrooms. After two minutes, move the skillet to the oven and bake until the frittata is completely cooked. Cut into 4 equal wedges and serve warm.

Sausage and Mushroom Strata (180 calories per serving)

Yields: 12 servings

Ingredients

- 2 tablespoons grated parmesan cheese
- Fresh ground pepper to taste
- ½ teaspoon paprika
- 1 cup sliced mushroom
- ½ cup green onion, chopped
- 12 ounces egg substitute
- 3 large eggs
- 4 ounces reduced-fat shredded sharp cheddar cheese
- 2 cups fat free milk
- 12 ounces turkey sausage
- 8 ounces wheat ciabatta bread, cut into 1-inch cubes

Instructions

Preheat oven to 400 degrees. On a baking sheet, arrange bread cubes and bake them at 400 degrees for about 8 minutes. Over medium-high heat, heat a medium skillet and add sausage to it. Cook until the sausage is brown, while stirring to crumble.

In a large mixing bowl, combine cheese, egg substitute, milk, salt, pepper and paprika and parmesan cheese. Whisk the mixture thoroughly. Add scallions, sausage, bread and mushrooms, tossing well to coat bread. Into a 13 inch by 9 inch baking dish, spoon the mixture, cover and refrigerate for about 8 hours.

Preheat oven to 350 degrees. Uncover casserole and bake at 350 degrees for 50 minutes. Cut into 12 pieces and serve immediately.

Pancakes with cream cheese topping (230 calories per serving)

Yields: 5 servings

Ingredients

- Pancakes:
- ½ teaspoon red paste food coloring
- 1 teaspoon vanilla
- 1 cup + 2 tablespoons fat-free milk
- 1 large egg
- ¼ cup sugar
- ¼ teaspoon salt
- ½ tablespoon unsweetened cocoa powder
- 2 ¼ teaspoons baking powder
- ½ cup unbleached all-purpose flour
- ½ cup white whole wheat flour
- Cream cheese topping:
- 1 tablespoon fat-free milk
- 3 tablespoons honey
- 3 tablespoon plain fat free yogurt
- 2 ounces 1/3 less fat cream cheese

Instructions

Combine the cream cheese topping ingredients and set aside. In a large bowl, mix baking powder, flours, sugar, cocoa powder and salt and set aside.

In a separate bowl, dissolve the food coloring with the milk and whisk in egg and vanilla.

Combine dry and wet ingredients until there are no more visible dry spots. Lightly coat a large griddle pan with oil and heat it on a medium-low heat. On it, pour ¼ cup of the pancake batter.

Flip the pancake when it starts to bubble and the edge begins to set. Do the same with the remaining batter.

Serve immediately by placing 2 pancakes on each plate then topping with about 2 ½ tablespoons of the cream cheese topping.

Granola (200 calories per serving)

Yields: 24 servings

Ingredients

- Cooking spray
- 1 cup raisins
- ¾ cup walnuts, chopped
- 2 cups bran flakes
- ½ cup unsweetened coconut, shredded
- 1 cup almonds, silvered
- 6 cups rolled oats (old fashioned)
- 1 ½ teaspoon vanilla
- 4 tablespoons honey
- ¼ cup canola oil

Instructions

Preheat oven to 325 degrees. In a small saucepan, place honey, vanilla and oil and cook gently over low heat while stirring for 5 minutes until combined.

In a large mixing bowl, place the remaining ingredients, apart from the raisins and mix properly. Stir in the oil-honey mixture ensuring that the grains are evenly coated. Using cooking oil, spray a baking tray then spread the cereal over it and put in the oven for 25 minutes. Stir occasionally to prevent the mixture from burning. Set it aside and allow it to cool. Add raisin and stir evenly through the mixture of the grain.

Overnight Oatmeal (240 calories per serving)

Yields: 4 servings

Ingredients

- 1 teaspoon cinnamon
- 1 teaspoon molasses
- 1/3 cup dried apricot, chopped
- 1/3 cup dried cherries
- 1/3 cup raisins
- 2 cups steel-cut oats
- 4 cups water
- 4 cups fat free milk

Instructions

Combine all the ingredients in a slow cooker and turn on heat to low. Cover the cooker with a lid and cook overnight for 9 hours. Serve by spooning into bowls and enjoy.

Breakfast Granola Bars (160 calories per serving)

Yields: 18 servings

Ingredients

- 1 teaspoon vanilla
- ½ cup peanut butter
- ½ cup light corn syrup
- ½ cup firmly packed brown sugar
- ½ cup raisins
- 2 cups old fashioned oatmeal
- 2 ½ cups toasted rice cereal

Instructions

In a large mixing bowl, combine oatmeal, rice cereal, and raisin and mix with a wooden spoon.

Mix corn syrup and brown sugar in a 1-quart saucepan and turn the heat to medium high. Bring the mixture to the boil by turning the heat to medium high. Remove the saucepan from the heat once it has boiled.

In a saucepan, stir a mixture of sugar, vanilla and peanut butter until very smooth. Pour this mixture in the bowl containing the raisin and cereal.

Into a 9 by 13 inch baking pan, press the mixture and let it cool completely before cutting it into 18 bars.

Serve and enjoy!

Breakfast Quinoa (320 calories per serving)

Yields: 4 servings

Ingredients

- ¼ cup almonds, sliced
- ¼ teaspoon cinnamon
- ¼ cup dried currants
- ¼ cup honey
- 1 cup uncooked and rinsed quinoa
- 2 cups non-fat milk

Instructions

In a medium saucepan, boil the milk. Add quinoa and return to boil. After 5 minutes, cover it, reduce the heat to medium –low then simmer for 15 minutes. Remove from the heat then add remaining ingredients.

Cover and leave it stand for about 15 minutes.

Serve.

Breakfast Pancakes (180 calories per serving)

Yields: 8 servings

Ingredients

- 1 teaspoon salt
- 1 teaspoon pumpkin pie spice
- 1 tablespoon baking powder
- 2 tablespoons brown sugar
- 2 cups flour
- 2 tablespoons vegetable oil
- 1¾ cups low-fat milk
- ½ cup canned pumpkin
- 1 egg

Instructions

In a large mixing bowl, combine eggs, oil, milk and pumpkin. Into this mixture add baking powder, salt, brown sugar and flour and stir gently.

Heat your skillet on medium heat then coat it lightly with cooking spray. Pour ¼ cup batter on the hot skillet. Cook until bubbles begin to burst and then flip over. Cook until it turns to golden brown. Do the same for the remaining batter.

Serve hot.

Broccoli and Cheese omelets (104 calories per serving)

Yields: 9 serving

Ingredients

- Cooking spray
- Salt and fresh pepper
- 1 tablespoon olive oil
- ¼ cup grated parmesan cheese
- ¼ cup reduced fat cheddar,
- 1 cup egg whites
- 4 whole eggs
- 4 cups broccoli florets

Instructions

Preheat oven to 350 degrees. Steam broccoli for about 7 minutes then mash into small pieces before adding olive oil, pepper and salt. Mix them well.

Spray cooking spray into muffin tin and divide the broccoli mixture evenly into 9 tins.

Whisk eggs, egg whites grated cheese, pepper and salt in a medium bowl. Pour this mixture into greased tins over broccoli until past ¾ full. Finish with cheddar and bake for 20 minutes.

Serve immediately.

Chapter 7: Dash Diet Main Dishes

In this section, we deal with main meals. These are healthy choices that use the correct ingredients to comply with the diet.

Apple Turkey Gyro (120 calories per serving)

Yields: 4 servings

Ingredients

- ½ cup low fat free plain yogurt
- 6 whole wheat pocket pita bread, warmed
- 1 golden delicious apple, cored and finely chopped
- ½ pound cooked turkey or chicken breasts, cut into thin strips
- 2 tablespoons lemon juice
- 1 cup sweet green pepper, thinly sliced
- 1 cup onion, sliced
- 1 tablespoon vegetable oil

Instructions

Put oil in a large skillet and heat it over medium heat. Add peppers, lemon juice and onion and cook until tender. Add turkey and apple to the skillet and stir. Leave it to cook until the turkey is soft enough.

In each pitta, fill with some of mixture, drizzle with yoghurt and then serve warm.

Caramelized onion and Asparagus frittata
(190 calories per serving)

Yields: 4 servings

Ingredients

- Fresh ground pepper to taste
- ½ teaspoon kosher salt
- ¼ cup plus 1 tablespoon parmesan cheese, grated
- 6 large eggs
- ¼ cup fresh basil, thinly sliced
- 3 green onions, sliced
- 2 cups (about 1 bunch) asparagus, cut into 1 inch sections
- 2 teaspoons balsamic vinegar
- 1 medium onion, thinly sliced
- 1 teaspoon olive oil

Instructions

Preheat the boiler to high.

Heat a 12 inch, ovenproof sauté pan over medium heat. Add onions and olive oil to it and cook until soft and slightly brown. To the onions, add balsamic vinegar and stir. Add the asparagus and two tablespoons of water then cover to steam it for four minutes while stirring occasionally.

In a medium mixing bowl, whisk eggs and stir in ¼ cup of the grated cheese, a few twists of fresh ground pepper and ¼ teaspoon of the kosher salt. Back to the cooked asparagus and onions, add the remaining ¼ teaspoon of kosher salt, green onions and basil then stir to combine.

To the same asparagus and onion mixture, add the egg mixture and mix slightly with a spatula. Pull the cooked egg from the bottom towards the top then allow the mixture to cook for more than 2 minutes over medium heat.

Put the pan under the pre-heated boiler until it is bubbled and browned slightly. Remove the pan from the broiler and sprinkle the remaining tablespoon cheese on it.

Serve the frittata after five minutes by slicing it into 4 wedges.

Sunshine Wrap (192 calories per serving)

Yields: 4 servings

Ingredients

- 4 large lettuce leaves, washed and patted dry
- 1 large whole wheat tortilla
- ¼ teaspoon black pepper
- ¼ teaspoon garlic powder
- 1 teaspoon soy sauce
- 2 tablespoons mayonnaise
- ¼ cup onion, minced
- 2/3 cup canned mandarin oranges, drained
- ½ cup celery, diced
- 8 ounces chicken breast

Instructions

Cook chicken breast in a non-stick pan on a medium-high heat until soft. Set aside and leave to cool enough to handle. Cut the breast into 4-inch cubes. Put the cubes, onions, oranges, and celery in a medium mixing bowl and mix them.

Add soy sauce, mayonnaise, pepper and garlic and mix gently until the chicken is evenly coated. Cut tortilla with clean kitchen scissors into 4 quarters. On top of each quarter, place a lettuce leaf and trim it to fit the shape of the tortilla.

Divide the chicken mixture into four and put each in the middle of each lettuce leaf. Roll the tortillas up into a cone with two straight edges coming together and the curved edges creating the opening of a cone.

Serve like a sandwich wrap.

Mushroom Mozzarella wraps (240 calories per serving)

Yields: 2 servings

Ingredients

- ¼ cup shredded part-skim mozzarella cheese
- 1 plum tomato, diced
- ½ pound fresh spinach, trimmed and steamed
- 2 whole wheat 8" tortillas
- 1 teaspoon minced garlic
- 8 ounces fresh mushrooms sliced
- 1 tablespoon olive oil

Instructions

Preheat oven to 350 degrees. On a sauté pan, heat 1 tablespoon olive oil over high heat.

Add to it a layer of garlic and mushrooms and let them sauté. Once the mushrooms turn to a reddish brown, turn them and leave to sauté until a similar color is achieved.

Lay flat tortillas leaves, on each, arrange layers of tomato, spinach and cooked mushrooms. Roll the tortilla leaves and place them on a slightly coated baking dish. Bake it for about 10 minutes.

Cut the tortillas crosswise into quarters and serve warm.

Salmon Salad Pita (180 calories per serving)

Yields: 3 servings

Ingredients

- 3 pieces of small whole wheat pit bread
- 3 lettuce leaves
- Black pepper to taste
- Pinch of dill, dried or fresh
- 1 teaspoon capers, rinsed and chopped
- 1 tablespoon red onion, minced
- 2 tablespoons red bell pepper, minced
- 1 tablespoon lemon juice
- 3 tablespoon plain fat-free yogurt
- ¾ cup canned salmon

Instructions

In a small mixing bowl, mix all ingredients except the bread and lettuce in order to make the salmon salad. Inside each pita, place 1 lettuce leaf and 1/3 cup salmon salad then serve hot.

Apple Swiss Panini (280 calories per serving)

Yields: 4 servings

Ingredients

- Cooking spray
- 1 cup arugula leaves
- 6 ounces low fat Swiss cheese, thinly sliced
- 2 crisp apples, thinly sliced
- ¼ cup non-fat honey mustard
- 8 slices whole-grain bread

Instructions

Preheat Panini press or non-stick skillet on medium heat then spread honey mustard over each slice of bread (ensure it is even).

Make layers of apple slices, arugula leaves and cheese over 4 slices of bread. Top each with slices of bread that have remained.

Slightly coat your skillet with cooking spray. Grill each sandwich until bread has toasted and all cheese melted. Allow pan to cool slightly before serving.

Tuna Melt (210 calories per serving)

Yields: 4 servings

Ingredients

- Salt and black pepper to taste
- 3 ounces reduced cheddar cheese, grated
- 2 whole-wheat English muffins split
- ¼ cup low fat Russian salad dressing
- ¼ cup chopped onion
- 1/3 cup chopped celery
- 6 ounces white tuna packed in water, drained

Instructions

Preheat broiler on medium heat. In a mixing bowl, combine onion, salad dressing, tuna and celery and season with pepper and salt and mix well.

Half the English muffins then on the baking sheet, place the side that is split up and top with ¼ of tuna mixture. Broil until heated through. Top with cheese before returning them to the broiler to melt the cheese.

Serve warm or at room temperature.

Grilled Veggie Sandwich (240 calories per serving)

Yields: 4 servings

Ingredients

- ½ cup crumbled reduced-fat feta cheese
- 2 slices focaccia bread
- 1 small yellow squash, sliced
- 1 red onion, sliced
- 1 small zucchini, sliced
- 1 cup red bell peppers sliced
- 1/8 cup olive oil
- 1 tablespoon lemon juice
- 3 cloves garlic, minced
- 3 tablespoons light mayonnaise

Instructions

Combine the garlic, lemon juice and mayonnaise in a mixing bowl and refrigerate.

Preheat the grill to high. Brush grate of grill and vegetables on both sides with olive oil. In the middle of grill, place bell peppers and zucchini then surround this with squash pieces and onion sets. Cook for 3 minutes on one side and do the same for the other side, then remove from the grill.

On the bread slices, spread a little mayonnaise and top up with cheese. Place the slices on the grill with the side with the cheese facing up. Cover the grill with a lid for about three minutes while watching the bottom side not to burn.

Layer the bread slices with vegetables after removing them from the grill.

Serve immediately and enjoy!

Tuna Salad (245 calories per serving)

Yields: 2 servings

Ingredients

- Black pepper to taste
- 1 tablespoon fresh parmesan cheese, shaved
- 2 cups arugula
- ¼ cup chopped green onion tops
- 1 tablespoon red wine vinegar
- 1 tablespoon extra-virgin olive oil
- 1 cup cooked pasta
- 1 (5 ounces) can light tuna in water, drained

Instructions

Toss tuna with olive oil, onion, vinegar, cooked pasta and arugula into a large mixing bowl and mix with a spatula.

Divide between two plates and top with cheese. Add pepper to taste.

Serve immediately.

Turkey and Cheese Sandwich (190 calories per serving)

Yields: 2 servings

Ingredients

- Pepper, coarsely ground
- ¼ cup shredded low fat mozzarella cheese
- 1 pear, cored and sliced
- 2 slices (1 ounces each) reduced-sodium cooked turkey
- 2 teaspoons Dijon-style mustard
- 2 slices multi-grain sandwich bread

Instructions

On each slice of bread, spread a tablespoon of mustard; arrange the pear slices onto this, followed by turkey slices. Sprinkle two tablespoons of cheese on each slice followed by pepper.

Broil the sandwich 5 inches from heat for about 3 minutes. Divide each sandwich into two then serve with the face open.

Rice Bowl (330 calories per serving)

Yields: 2 servings

Ingredients

- 2 tablespoons low fat sour cream
- 2 tablespoons shredded cheese
- 4 tablespoons salsa
- 1 cup cooked brown rice
- 1 cup cooked meat, chopped and shredded
- 1 cup mixture of chopped onion, tomato, corn, zucchini and bell pepper
- 1 teaspoon vegetable oil

Instructions

Put vegetable oil in a medium skillet and heat it over medium high heat. Add vegetables to the skillet and simmer for about 4 minutes. Add cooked rice and cooked meat then heat the mixture all through.

Divide the mixture into 2 and top each bowl with cheese, salsa, and sour cream.

Serve warm and enjoy.

Guacamole with Black Bean Cake (170 calories per serving)

Yields: 4 servings

Ingredients

- 1 small plum tomato
- 1 tablespoon lime juice
- ½ medium avocado, seeded and peeled
- 1 large egg
- 1 teaspoon ground cumin
- 1 (7-ounce) can chipotle in adobo sauce
- 1 (15- ounce) can low sodium black beans, rinsed and drained
- 2 cloves garlic
- 2 tablespoons fresh cilantro
- 2 slices whole wheat bread, torn

Instructions

In a blender, place torn pieces of bread and process it to coarse crumbs. Put it in a bowl and set aside. In the same blender, add garlic and cilantro and process until they are finely chopped. Add cumin, a teaspoon of adobo sauce, 1 chipotle pepper and beans. Process until the desired smoothness is achieved.

Add the mixture to the crumbs of bread then add the egg and mix properly. Shape the mixture into 4 patties that are half inch thick. Lightly grease the grill rack. Grill the patties uncovered over medium heat for about 10 minutes.

In a separate small bowl, mash avocado and stir in lime juice then sprinkle with pepper and salt to obtain your guacamole.

Serve the patties with tomato and guacamole.

Veggie quesadillas with yogurt (240 calories per serving)

Yields: 4 servings

Ingredients

- 1 medium carrot, shredded
- 6 soft corn tortillas
- 1 cup low-fat shredded cheese
- ½ cup corn kernels
- ½ bell pepper, finely chopped
- 2 tablespoons cilantro, chopped
- 1 cup black beans
- ½ jalapeno pepper, finely diced

Yogurt dip:

- 2 tablespoons cilantro, chopped
- 1 cup plain non-fat yogurt
- Juice from ½ of lime

Instructions

Over low heat, preheat skillet. Set aside 3 tortillas and divide cilantro, beans, shredded carrot, peppers, corn and cheese between them. Cover each of the three tortillas with the remaining second tortillas.

Place a tortilla on a preheated dry skillet and warm until the tortilla is slightly brown and all cheese melted. Flip it over and make the other side slightly golden too.

Mix nonfat yogurt, lime juice, cilantro, and the nonfat yoghurt in a small bowl. Cut the quesadilla into 12 wedges (4 wedges on each).

Serve 3 wedges and ¼ cup of dip per person.

Refrigerate leftovers within 2 hours.

Shepherd pie (320 calories per serving)

Yields: 6 servings

Ingredients

- Ground pepper to taste
- ½ cup shredded cheddar cheese
- ¾ cup reduced sodium beef broth
- 4 cups frozen mixed vegetables
- 2 tablespoons flour
- 1 clove garlic, minced
- 1 medium onion, chopped
- 1 pound lean ground beef
- ½ cup low-fat milk
- 2 large baking potatoes, peeled and diced

Instructions

Bring to boil diced potatoes, water and barley in a saucepan. Reduce the heat and simmer for about 15 minutes.

Drain water from the potatoes, add milk and mash then set aside the mixture. Preheat the oven to 375 degrees. In a large greasy skillet, add onion, garlic and meat and cook on a low heat until everything is brown. Add in flour and cook for 1 minute while stirring.

Add vegetables and broth and cook for 5 minutes while stirring until bubbly. Into an 8 by 8inch baking dish, spoon vegetable mixture. Spread potato mixture over it. Sprinkle cheese on top and bake for 25 minutes until hot and bubbly.

Refrigerate leftovers within 3 hours.

Spaghetti Squash Lasagna (291 calories per serving)

Yields: 4 servings

Ingredients

- Ground red pepper to taste
- 6 ounces part-skim shredded mozzarella
- 8 teaspoon grated parmesan cheese
- 1 cup part-skim ricotta
- 3 cups roasted spaghetti squash
- 2 cups marinara sauce

Instructions

Roast spaghetti squash by cutting the squash into halves and scoop out the fibers and seeds with a spoon. Place on a baking sheet with the cut side up then sprinkle with pepper and salt to taste. Bake on the oven at 350 degrees until the skin gives easily when under pressure and the inside becomes tender.

Remove from the oven and set aside for 10 minutes. Scrape off the squash flesh a little at a time using a fork to separate spaghetti like strands. Measure 3 cups of lasagna recipe.

Preheat oven to 375 degrees.

At the bottom of a baking dish, spread marina sauce, followed by roasted spaghetti evenly spread and another layer of ricotta cheese. Sprinkle with ½ of mozzarella and parmesan. Add the remaining sauce and finish with the remaining mozzarella and parmesan. Cover the dish with foil and bake until the edges begin to bubble and all the cheese melted. Remove the cover and cook for five more minutes.

Remove from the oven and set aside to cool before serving.

Stuffed Poblano peppers (300 calories per serving)

Yields: 4 servings

Ingredients

- ½ cup Mexican blend cheese, shredded
- Freshly ground black pepper to taste
- 1/8 teaspoon cayenne pepper
- 1 teaspoon chili powder
- 1 teaspoon cumin
- 1 ½ cups frozen corn
- 1 (15-ounce) can black beans
- 1 ½ cup fresh grilled salsa
- ½ cup uncooked brown rice
- 4 large poblano peppers

Instructions

Boil water and bring rice to cook. Slice each poblano into halves and remove the ribs and seeds. In a baking dish, place the peppers and broil for about 4 minutes. Flip the peppers and broil for another 4 minutes. Be careful not to over burn the peppers.

Rinse and drain the black beans. Combine cayenne, chili powder, cumin, ¼ cup of cheese, corn salsa, beans, and pepper to taste in a large microwave safe bowl. In the microwave, heat the filling for about 3 minutes, stirring at intervals of 30 seconds.

Into each pepper half, spoon the filling and top up with the remaining cheese. Broil until all the cheese is melted.

Serve immediately.

Chapter 8: Dash Diet Dessert and Snack Recipes

This section is devoted to both snacks and desserts and may be the right place to look if you have a sweet tooth, or tend to eat between meals.

Apple-berry cobbler (136 calories per serving)

Yields: 6 servings

Ingredients

For the filling

- 1 ½ tablespoon cornstarch
- 2 teaspoons lemon juice
- 1 teaspoon lemon zest
- ½ teaspoon ground cinnamon
- 2 tablespoons brown sugar
- 2 cups chopped apples
- 1 cup fresh blueberries
- 1 cup fresh raspberries

Toppings:

- ¾ cup whole- wheat pastry flour
- 1 ½ tablespoons brown sugar
- ½ teaspoon vanilla
- ¼ teaspoon salt

- ¼ cup soy milk
- 1 egg white

Instructions

Preheat oven to 350 degrees F. Coat lightly 6 ovenproof ramekins with cooking spray.

Add lemon juice, lemon zest, cinnamon, sugar, apples, blueberries and raspberries in a medium mixing bowl and stir to obtain an even mixture. Add the cornstarch then stir until all the starch dissolves. Set this bowl aside.

Whisk egg whites in a separate bowl until lightly beaten. Add pastry flour, sugar, vanilla, salt and soy milk then stir to mix well.

Into the ramekins, divide the berry mixture equally then pour the toppings over each dish. Place the dishes in the oven on a large baking pan. Bake until the toppings are golden brown and berries tender.

Serve warm.

Creamy fruit dessert (154 calories per serving)

Yields: 4 servings

Ingredients

- 4 tablespoons shredded coconut toasted
- 1 can (8 ounces) water-packed pineapple chunks, drained
- 1 can (8.25 ounces) water-packed sliced peaches, drained
- 1 can (11 ounces) mandarin oranges, drained
- ½ teaspoon vanilla
- 1 teaspoon sugar
- ½ cup plain fat-free yogurt
- 4 ounces fat-free cream cheese, softened.

Instructions

Combine vanilla, sugar, cheese cream and yogurt in a small bowl and stir until it mixes evenly. Set the bowl aside.

Combine pineapple, oranges, and peaches in a separate bowl. Add cheese and cream mixture and mix. Put in the refrigerator covered until it is well chilled

Set four serving bowls and transfer the mixture then garnish with shredded coconut then serve immediately.

Fruitcake (229 calories per serving)

Yields: 12 servings

Ingredients

- ½ cup crushed walnuts
- 1 egg
- ½ teaspoon baking soda
- 1 cup whole-wheat pastry flour
- ½ cup oat flour
- ¼ cup milled flax
- ¼ cup sugar
- 2 tablespoons vanilla
- ½ cup apple juice
- Zest and juice of 1 lemon
- ½ teaspoon baking powder
- Zest and juice of one medium orange
- ½ cup crushed pineapple
- ½ cup unsweetened applesauce.

Instructions

Combine vanilla, fruit zests and juices, pineapple, applesauce and dried fruit in a medium brown and soak for about 20 minutes.

Combine baking powder, baking soda, pastry flour, oat flour, milled flax and sugar in a large bowl and stir to mix evenly. Pour the liquid and fruit mixture into the dry ingredients and stir to combine.

Line a loaf pan with baking paper and pour mixture into the pan. Bake for one hour at 325 degrees F. Leave the fruit cake to rest for 30 minutes.

Remove it from the pan and serve.

Orange dream (8 calories per serving)

Yields: 4 servings

Ingredients

- 4 peeled orange segments
- 5 ice cubes
- ½ teaspoon vanilla extract
- 1 teaspoon grated orange zest
- 1 tablespoon dark honey
- 1/3 cup soft tofu
- 1 cup light vanilla soy milk, chilled
- 1 ½ cups orange juice, chilled

Instructions

Combine ice cubes, vanilla, orange zest, honey, tofu, soy milk and orange juice in a blender and process until frothy and smooth.

Serve in 4 tall glasses and garnish each with an orange segment.

Tasty muffins (180 calories per serving)

Yields: 12 servings

Ingredients

- ½ teaspoon salt
- ½ teaspoon baking soda
- 1 teaspoon baking powder
- 1 teaspoon cinnamon
- 1 cup old-fashioned oatmeal
- 1½ cups flour
- 1 teaspoon vanilla
- ½ cup toasted walnuts
- ½ cup raisins
- ½ cup grated carrots
- 2 tablespoons vegetable oil
- 1/3 cup sugar
- 1 cup low fat milk
- 1 egg, beaten
- Nonstick cooking spay

Instructions

Preheat oven to 400 degrees. Use nonstick cooking spray to coat muffin tins.

In a mixing bowl, combine vanilla, walnuts, raisins, carrots, oil, sugar, milk and the egg. Mix evenly.

Mix baking powder, baking soda, salt, oatmeal and cinnamon in a separate bowl. Add wet ingredients to the dry ingredients and stir gently to moisten flour.

Fill muffin cups ¾ full and bake for 15 minutes.

Potato Nachos (192 calories per serving)

Yields: 5 servings

Ingredients

- ¾ cup salsa
- 1 tablespoon cilantro, chopped
- 1 cucumber, peeled and diced
- 1 medium tomato, diced ¾ cup
- 1 cup lettuce, shredded
- ½ cup cheddar cheese, shredded
- ½ teaspoon chili powder
- 8 ounces ground turkey, 99% fat free
- 2 teaspoons oil
- 1 pound small red potatoes, skin on

Instructions

Slice potatoes into ¼-inch thick circles. Coat the slices with oil lightly then arrange them on a baking sheet in 1 layer. Put them into the oven and bake for 30 minutes.

On a skillet, add chili powder and turkey and cook over medium heat until the turkey turns golden brown.

Transfer the potatoes from the oven to an oven safe dish, then top with turkey and sprinkle with cheese. Put the dish in the oven to melt the cheese.

Remove the dish from the oven and top with salsa, cilantro, cucumber, tomato and lettuce.

Serve immediately.

Lemon Smoothie (190 calories per serving)

Yields: 1 serving

Ingredients

- Lemon zest for garnish
- ½ teaspoon finely grated lemon zest
- 1 teaspoon fresh lemon juice
- 2 tablespoons granulated sugar
- 1 container (6 oz.) plain fat-free yoghurt
- 3 milk ice cubes, cracked

Instructions

Make milk ice cubes by filling an ice cube tray with non-fat milk and freeze until solid. Thereafter, combine all ingredients in a blender, including the cubes and process on high until desired consistency is achieved.

Serve immediately in a tall glass and garnish with the lemon zest.

Green smoothie (350 calories per serving)

Yields: 1 serving

Ingredients

- ¼ cup plain non-fat yogurt
- 1 cup baby spinach, packed
- 1 medium banana, peeled and frozen
- ½ teaspoon vanilla
- ½ cup fat free milk
- ¾ cup frozen mango
- ¼ cup whole oats

Instructions

Put yogurt, milk and oats in a blender and run it on a high for 15 seconds. Add the remaining ingredients and process them together until the required consistency is achieved. Serve immediately in a glass and enjoy!

Berry Blast (150 calories per serving)

Yields: 4 serving

Ingredients

- 1 cup blueberries, rinsed
- 1 cup low- fat granola
- 1 cup strawberries, rinsed and sliced
- 1 cup plain, low-fat yogurt

Instructions

Set out 4 glasses and in each, divide the strawberries equally. Sprinkle granola over the berries in the glasses. On top of the granola, add the blueberries. Finish by spooning the yogurt on top of the blueberries and enjoy.

Berry Muesli (170 calories per serving)

Yields: 4 servings

Ingredients

- ¼ cup walnuts, chopped and toasted
- ½ cup frozen blueberries
- ½ cup chopped apple
- ½ cup dried fruit, either, raisins, apricots or dates
- ½ cup non-fat milk
- A pinch of salt
- 1 cup of fruit yogurt
- 1 cup old-fashioned rolled oats (raw)

Instructions

Mix oats, milk, yogurt and salt in a medium bowl then cover it and refrigerate for about 12 hours. Set aside and add the dried and fresh fruit. Mix them gently.

In small separate dishes, serve scopes of muesli and sprinkle each serving with chopped nuts. In case of left overs, refrigerate within 2-3 hours.

Pumpkin cookies (93 calories per serving)

Yields: 48 servings

Ingredients

- 1 cup walnuts, chopped
- 1 cup raisins
- ½ teaspoon salt
- 1 ½ teaspoons pumpkin pie spice mix
- 1 tablespoon baking powder
- 1¼ cups whole wheat flour
- 1½ cups flour
- ½ cup vegetable oil
- 2 eggs
- 1½ cups brown sugar
- 1¾ cups cooked, pureed pumpkin

Instructions

Preheat oven to 400 degrees. In a mixing bowl, add eggs, pumpkin, oil and brown sugar. Process all the dry ingredients in a blender and add them to the pumpkin mixture. Add raisins and nuts.

On the greased cookie sheet, drop a teaspoon sized cookie each 1 inch apart. Flatten each cookie with your hand or use the bottom of a glass. Bake until golden brown then serve.

Chapter 9: DASH Salad Recipes

In this chapter, I have highlighted some exciting DASH salad recipes for you to try out. These will definitely help you lose weight and meet the calorie requirements.

Almond Chicken Pear salad (232 calories per serving)

Yields: 8 servings

Ingredients

- 4 cups of cooked skinless and boneless, chicken breasts
- ½ cup celery, diced finely
- 1 cup green pepper, sliced thinly
- ½ teaspoon salt
- 4 tablespoons mayonnaise (reduced calories)
- 1 teaspoon mustard
- 1 cup low-fat plain yogurt
- ½ teaspoon ground ginger
- 1 Lettuce
- 4 fresh pears
- 4 tablespoons of toasted and slivered almonds

Instructions

First, take the chicken breasts and dice them into ½ inch cubes. Keep aside.

Next, wash the pears well. Cut them in halves and remove the cores and seeds. Cut the pears into smaller pieces and keep aside.

Wash the lettuce well and arrange the leaves neatly to serve the salad on.

Toss the chopped celery, green pepper and chicken together in a large bowl. Sprinkle the salt on top of the mixture. Combine well.

Take a small bowl. Add the mustard, mayonnaise, ginger and yogurt to the bowl and mix well. Add the paste to the chicken mixture and mix well.

Finally, add in the pears and mix well.

Distribute the salad evenly among the lettuce leaves. Sprinkle the slivered almonds on top of the salad. Serve immediately.

Cucumber and Radish Salad with Farro (170 calories per serving)

Yields: 4 servings

Ingredients:

- 3 cucumbers
- 1 cup faro
- ¼ cup of mint leaves, finely chopped
- 1 bunch of radishes
- 2 cloves of garlic, finely minced
- 3 tablespoons of fresh lemon juice
- 2 tablespoons of olive oil
- Freshly ground black pepper
- 3 teaspoons of white wine vinegar
- Pinch of salt
- ¼ cup of fresh dill, finely chopped
- 2 ounces of feta cheese (reduced fat)

Instructions:

Read the instructions on the package and prepare the faro accordingly. It should be cooked in approximately 30 to 45 minutes. Please note that the faro is cooked when it is tender and not when it is falling apart. Once it is cooked through, drain it. Rinse with cool water and drain the water again. Transfer the rinsed faro to a clean and large bowl and keep aside.

Wash the cucumbers and radishes well. Peel their skins and slice them thinly. Add the sliced cucumbers and radishes to the cooked faro and mix well.

Now, add the lemon juice, vinegar, garlic, salt and pepper to the bowl and mix well. Drizzle with olive oil and toss the contents of the bowl well. Next, add the chopped dill and mint to the bowl. Finally, add the cheese to the bowl and toss well. Serve immediately.

Fiesta Bean Salad

Yields: 8 servings

Ingredients:

- 2 15 ounces cans of low-sodium black beans
- 6 tablespoons of fresh lime juice
- 2 tablespoons of extra-virgin olive oil
- 2 teaspoons of cumin
- 2 pinches of crushed red pepper flakes
- 2 cups of canned chickpeas
- 2 cups of cherry tomatoes, cut into halves
- ½ cup of red onion, finely chopped
- ½ cup of fresh cilantro, finely chopped
- 2 medium avocadoes
- 4 cloves garlic, finely minced

Instructions:

Ensure that the black beans and chickpeas are rinsed and drained well. Keep aside.

Take the avocadoes and peel their skins off. Cut in halves and remove the pits. Dice it finely and keep aside.

Take a small bowl. Add the lime juice, olive oil, red pepper flakes, garlic and cumin to it and mix well.

Take a large bowl. Add the black beans, tomatoes, onions, chickpeas and cilantro to the bowl and mix well. Add the lime juice dressing to the bowl and mix well.

Add in the avocadoes before serving.

Barley summer salad (150 calories per serving)

Yields: 20 servings

Ingredients:

- 4 cups of apples, deseeded and chopped into smaller pieces
- 6 cups of water
- ½ cup of dried cranberries
- 2 cups of dry barley
- 2 cups of fresh blueberries
- 2 cups of sweet snap peas
- 1 cup of green onions, thinly sliced
- 1 cup of red bell pepper, finely chopped
- 2 tablespoons of vinegar
- 6 tablespoons of vegetable oil
- ½ cup of lemon or lime juice

Instructions:

Take a medium saucepan. Add the barley and water to it and bring it to a boil. Once the water starts boiling, turn down the heat. Cover the lid of the saucepan and cook the barley for at least 45 minutes. At the end of 45 minutes, drain the hot water from the saucepan. Add cold water to the pan and rinse the barley well. Drain the cold water and transfer the barley to a large bowl.

Add the apples, snap peas, onions and red bell pepper to the bowl. Mix well.

Now, add the cranberries, blueberries, vinegar and vegetable oil to the bowl and mix well.

Finally, pour the lemon juice over the contents of the bowl. Mix well. Serve immediately.

Apricot Pasta Salad with chicken (360 calories per serving)

Yields: 8 servings

Ingredients:

For the Dressing

- 4 apricots, peeled and quartered
- 4 tablespoons of white wine vinegar
- ½ teaspoon of salt
- 2 tablespoons of sugar
- 6 tablespoons of olive oil
- 2 tablespoons of finely chopped fresh basil

For the Salad

- ½ lb fusilli pasta
- 12 fresh apricots, peeled and quartered
- 4 cups of low sodium chicken broth
- 4 skinless and boneless chicken breasts
- 2 red bell peppers, sliced thinly into long strips
- 4 small zucchini ends (trimmed), halved
- 2 tablespoons of fresh basil, finely chopped
- 2 cups of the apricot basil dressing

Instructions:

Add the apricots, salt, sugar and white wine vinegar to the bowl of a blender. Pulse the contents of the blender till they mix well. As the blender is running, pour in the olive oil slowly. This will ensure that the mixture turns smooth and thick. Once the olive oil is mixed in, add the fresh basil to the blender and mix well. Keep the dressing aside.

Take a medium sized saucepan. Add the chicken broth to the pan and heat it. Once the broth begins to boil, reduce the heat and allow it to simmer. Now, add the chicken breasts to the pan. Cover the lid of the pan and allow the breasts to simmer in the broth for at least six minutes. This should give enough time for the chicken to cook through thoroughly. At the end of six minutes, remove the breasts from the broth. Allow the breasts to cool down and shred it into smaller pieces, with the help of a fork.

Read the instructions on the package and cook the pasta. Drain and allow the pasta to cool and transfer to a large bowl. Add the chicken, apricots, red peppers, zucchini and basil to the bowl and mix well. Add the salad dressing to the bowl and mix well. Serve immediately.

Black Bean and Corn Salsa Salad (190 calories per serving)

Yields: 16 servings

Ingredients:

For the Dressing

- ½ cup of fresh lime juice
- 2 cloves of garlic, finely minced
- 2/3 cups of olive oil
- 1 teaspoon of ground coriander
- 1 teaspoon of ground cumin

For the Salad

- 4 cups of cooked black beans
- 4 cups of corn kernels
- 1 ½ cups of red bell pepper, deseeded and chopped finely
- 1 ½ cups of orange bell pepper, deseeded and chopped finely
- 4 small jalapeno chilies, deseeded and finely minced
- 1 ½ cups of sweet white or red onions, chopped finely
- 2 large ripe tomatoes, chopped finely
- 1 cup of fresh parsley or cilantro, chopped finely

Instructions:

Take a small bowl. Add the olive oil, minced garlic, lime juice, cumin and coriander to it. Whisk well. Keep aside for thirty minutes to ensure that the flavors blend well.

Take a large bowl. Add the corn kernels, black beans, jalapenos, onion and bell peppers to the bowl and mix well.

Add the dressing to the salad and mix well. Add the tomato pieces to the salad and mix well.

Cover the bowl and keep it in the refrigerator for few hours. This will give enough time for the flavors to blend.

Add the chopped parsley or cilantro to the salad before serving.

Mediterranean Quinoa salad (200 calories per serving)

Yields: 12 servings

Ingredients:

- 2 cups of uncooked quinoa
- 4 cups of water
- ½ cup of red onion
- Juice from 1 lemon
- ½ cup kalamata olives, pitted and sliced thinly
- 4 tablespoons of extra virgin olive oil
- 2 cucumbers
- 2 cups of cherry tomatoes
- ½ cup of crumbled feta
- 4 teaspoons of black pepper
- Salt, to taste

Instructions:

Rinse the quinoa in water well for around 2 minutes.

Take a medium sized pot. Add the water to it. Add the rinsed quinoa and salt to the pot. Bring the contents of the pot to a boil. When the water begins to boil, reduce the heat to low. Cover the lid of the pot and allow its contents to simmer for around 15 minutes. At the end of 15 minutes, remove the pot from the heat. Let it rest in the pot, with the lid covered, for another five minutes. Transfer the cooked quinoa to a large bowl and keep it aside for cooling.

As the quinoa is cooling, wash the cucumbers well. Peel their skins off and dice them into smaller pieces. Keep aside. Dice the other vegetables finely.

Add the diced vegetables and olives to the cooled quinoa in the large bowl and toss well.

Pour the lemon juice on top of the contents of the bowl and mix well.

Drizzle olive oil over the salad and mix well.

Add the crumbled feta and pepper to the bowl and mix well. Serve immediately.

Quinoa fruit salad (220 calories per serving)

Yields: 12 servings

Ingredients:

- 2 cups of uncooked quinoa
- 4 cups of water
- 1 teaspoon salt

For the Honey Lime Dressing

- Juice from 2 large limes
- 6 tablespoons of honey
- 4 tablespoons of fresh mint, finely chopped

For the fruit

- 3 cups of blueberries
- 3 cups of strawberries, sliced thinly
- 3 cups of finely chopped mangoes
- ½ cup of goats cheese, crumbled

Instructions:

Rinse the quinoa in water well for around 2 minutes.

Take a medium sized pot. Add the water to it. Add the rinsed quinoa and salt to the pot. Bring the contents of the pot to a boil. When the water begins to boil, reduce the heat to low. Cover the lid of the pot and allow its contents to simmer for around 15 minutes. At the end of 15 minutes, remove the pot from the heat. Let it rest in the pot, with the lid covered, for another five minutes. Transfer the cooked quinoa to a large bowl and keep it aside for cooling.

As the quinoa is cooling, prepare the honey lime dressing. Take a medium bowl. Add the honey, lime juice and chopped mint to the bowl and mix well.

Add the blueberries, mangoes, cheese and strawberries to the cooled quinoa in the large bowl and toss well.

Pour the honey lime dressing on top of the contents of the bowl and mix well. Serve immediately.

Cherry and wild rice salad (261 calories per serving)

Yields: 12 servings

Ingredients:

- ½ cup of orange juice
- ½ teaspoon salt
- 1 teaspoon of orange zest
- 4 tablespoons of shallot, finely minced
- 2 tablespoons of balsamic vinegar
- ½ cup of extra-virgin olive oil
- 6 cups of cooked wild rice
- 2 teaspoons of Dijon mustard
- 2 cups of fresh sweet cherries, pits removed and cut in halves
- 1 ½ cups of celery, finely diced
- ½ cup of pecans, toasted and coarsely chopped
- 1 cup of dried tart cherries, chopped roughly
- ½ cup of flat leaf parsley, finely chopped

Instructions:

First, let's get started with the vinaigrette. Take a large bowl. Add the orange juice, zest and salt to it and mix well. Now, add the minced shallot and vinegar to the bowl and mix well. Allow the mixture to rest for five minutes. This should give enough time for the shallots to mellow down. At the end of five minutes, add the extra virgin olive oil and Dijon mustard to the bowl and whisk well.

Add the cooked wild rice to the bowl followed by the cherries. Add the pecans, celery and parsley to the bowl and mix well. Keep mixing till the vinaigrette is distributed evenly. Serve immediately.

Strawberry, shrimp and feta salad (270 calories per serving)

Yields: 8 servings

Ingredients:

For the vinaigrette

- ½ teaspoon salt
- 4 tablespoons of water
- 6 tablespoons of extra virgin olive oil
- 4 tablespoons of balsamic vinegar
- ½ teaspoon black pepper

For the salad

- 1 ½ pounds of raw shrimp, peeled and deveined
- 4 cups of strawberries, stems removed and cut in quarters
- 2/3 cups of red onions, thinly sliced
- 4 ounces of feta cheese, crumbled
- 16 cups of watercress and chopped butter lettuce
- 2 cucumbers, sliced thinly

Instructions:

First, take a small bowl. Add the balsamic vinegar, olive oil, water, pepper and salt to it and whisk well. Keep aside.

Take a large bowl. Add the onions to it. Pour around 2 tablespoons of the vinaigrette on top of it and mix well. Let it rest for five minutes. This will give enough time for the onions to mellow.

Arrange the shrimps neatly on a charcoal grill or a grill pan on stove top. Grill them for around five minutes. Cook till both the sides are pink and completely cooked.

Take another small bowl. Add the strawberries and two tablespoons of the vinaigrette to it and toss well.

Add the watercress and butter lettuce to the bowl containing the onions. Pour the remaining vinaigrette on top of the contents of the bowl and mix well. Divide the greens and onions among 8 plates. Arrange the shrimps and strawberries neatly on top of the greens. Garnish the salad with the crumbled feta cheese and arrange the cucumber slices neatly. Serve immediately.

Southwest black bean salad (90 calories per serving)

Yields: 13 servings

Ingredients:

- 1 medium tomato, coarsely chopped
- 15.5 ounces can of black beans
- 1/3 cup of red onion, finely chopped
- 1 scallion, finely chopped
- 9 ounces of cooked corn
- Juice from 2 limes
- 1 tablespoon of olive oil
- 1 teaspoon of salt
- 2 tablespoons of fresh cilantro, finely minced
- 1 teaspoon of fresh black pepper
- ½ avocado
- ¼ cup of cotija cheese
- 1 jalapeno, diced finely

Instructions:

Ensure that the black beans are rinsed with water and drained well.

Peel the skins off the avocado and cut in halves. Remove the pit. Dice one half of the avocado into smaller pieces.

Take a large bowl. Add the black beans, tomato, corn, scallion, salt, onion, pepper and cilantro to the bowl and mix well. Pour the lemon juice on top of the contents of the bowl and mix well. Stir in the olive oil and mix well.

Place the bowl in the refrigerator and allow its contents to marinate at least for thirty minutes.

At the end of 30 minutes, remove the bowl from the refrigerator and divide it among 13 bowls. Add the diced avocado and cheese to the salad. Serve immediately.

Mixed greens salad with blue cheese, chicken and strawberries with poppy seed dressing (290 calories per serving)

Yields: 8 servings

Ingredients:

For the dressing

- 2 tablespoons of red wine vinegar
- 2 tablespoons of cider vinegar
- 4 tablespoons of olive oil
- 2 teaspoons of finely minced shallots
- 3 tablespoons of honey
- 1 tablespoon of poppy seeds

For the salad

- 10 ounces of mixed baby greens
- ½ cup of thinly slivered almonds
- 4 cups of strawberries, thinly sliced
- ½ cup of blue cheese
- 24 ounces of grilled chicken, sliced thinly

Instructions:

First, let's get started with the preparation of the dressing. Take a small bowl. Add the red wine vinegar, olive oil, cider vinegar, shallots, poppy seeds and honey to it and mix well.

Take a large bowl. Add the baby greens, strawberries, chicken slices to it and mix well. Add the almonds and blue cheese to the bowl and toss well.

Pour the dressing on top of the salad and toss well. Ensure that the dressing is distributed well. Divide the salad evenly among 8 serving bowls and serve immediately.

Tuna and Potato Salad (216 calories per serving)

Yields: 8 servings

Ingredients:

- 2 6-ounce cans of white tuna in water, rinsed and drained
- 24 steamed asparagus spears
- 16 small red potatoes
- 16 radishes
- 4 tablespoons of finely minced red onions
- 18 Kalamata olives, pits removed and cut in halves
- 6 tablespoons of red wine vinegar
- 8 teaspoons of olive oil
- 4 tablespoons of fresh parsley, finely chopped
- Black pepper, to taste
- Salt, to taste
- Water

Instructions:

Ensure that the potatoes are washed well. Cut the potatoes in quarters and transfer it to a large pot. Pour enough water into the pot and place it on high heat. Allow the water to boil for at least 10 minutes. This is enough time for the potatoes to turn tender. At the end of ten minutes, remove the pot from the heat and drain the water.

Place the cooked potatoes neatly on a large platter. Arrange the tuna, onion, olives, radishes and asparagus on the platter neatly.

Take a small bowl. Add the olive oil, parsley and vinegar to the bowl and whisk well.

Drizzle vinaigrette over the salad. Sprinkle the salt and black pepper on top of the salad. Serve immediately.

Panzanella salad (94 calories per serving)

Yields: 8 servings

Ingredients:

- 1 cup of cucumber, deseeded and diced finely
- ½ red onion, finely chopped
- 8 to 10 medium tomatoes
- 8 to 10 basil leaves, chopped coarsely
- Extra-virgin olive oil spray
- 1 tablespoon of extra-virgin olive oil
- 6 ounces of whole wheat French bread
- ¼ teaspoon salt
- ¼ teaspoon pepper

Instructions:

Wash the tomatoes well. Dice them into one inch cubes.

Spray the wheat bread lightly with olive oil spray and place it on a grill. Grill it over medium heat till the bread is nicely browned and toasted. Once it is toasted well, remove the bread from the heat. Cut into 1 inch cubes.

Take a large bowl. Add the chopped tomatoes, onion, basil, cucumber to the bowl and mix well. Add the olive oil, pepper and salt to the bowl next and mix well. Allow the mixture to rest for 30 minutes. This should be sufficient time for the flavors to blend well.

At the end of 30 minutes, add the bread cubes to the bowl and toss well. Divide it equally among 8 serving bowls and serve immediately.

Orange rice salad (200 calories per serving)

Yields: 14 servings

Ingredients:

- 1 cup of celery, washed and diced thinly
- 1 ½ cups of raisins
- 4 cups of brown rice, cooked and cooled
- 4 tablespoons of canola oil
- ½ cup of chopped nuts
- 2 tablespoons of orange juice
- ½ cup of fresh parsley, chopped finely
- 6 green onions, washed and sliced thinly
- 2 cans of mandarin oranges (with juice)
- Black Pepper, to taste

Instructions:

Take a medium sized bowl. Add the brown rice, diced celery and onions to the bowl and mix well.

Now, add the chopped nuts, raisins, mandarin oranges to the bowl and mix well.

Pour the orange juice and canola oil on top of the contents of the bowl. Garnish with chopped parsley and black pepper and mix well.

Place the bowl in the refrigerator for around one hour. This should be sufficient time for the flavors to blend together. At the end of one hour, remove the bowl from the refrigerator. Divide the salad equally among 14 bowls and serve immediately.

Pasta salad with arugula and walnut pesto (275 calories per serving)

Yields: 8 servings

Ingredients:

- 2 cups of arugula
- 4 cups of whole wheat pasta
- 1 cup of fat free Greek yogurt
- ¼ cup of walnuts
- ¼ cup of low fat mozzarella cheese
- Pepper, to taste
- 2 cloves of garlic
- Pinch of nutmeg
- Olive oil (for drizzling)
- ½ cup of sliced sun dried tomatoes
- Water

Instructions:

Take a large pot. Add the pasta to it. Pour enough water and bring it to a boil. Once the pasta is boiled well, drain the hot water. Transfer the cooked pasta to a large bowl and keep it aside.

Add the yogurt, walnuts, cheese, arugula, garlic and pepper to the bowl of a food processor. Pulse the contents till the consistency of the mixture is smooth and creamy. Add some more yogurt if the mixture is too thick.

Mix the pesto sauce with the cooked pasta. Keep folding till the pasta is completely coated with the pesto sauce. Divide the pasta among 8 serving bowls.

Drizzle with olive oil. Garnish with the sun dried tomatoes. Serve immediately.

Quinoa and fresh strawberry salad with goat cheese (290 calories per serving)

Yields: 6 servings

Ingredients:

- 1 ½ cups of quinoa
- 3 cups of water
- 3 cups of spinach, stems removed and cut into thin strips
- ¼ cup of sunflower seeds, roasted
- 1 ½ cups of strawberries, cut in quarters
- 3 ounces of goat cheese, crumbled

For the Balsamic Dressing

- 1 ½ tablespoons of olive oil
- 2 tablespoons of balsamic vinegar
- 1 teaspoon of honey

Instructions:

Rinse the quinoa well in water for around 2 minutes.

Take a medium sized pot. Add the water to it. Add the rinsed quinoa and salt to the pot. Bring the contents of the pot to a boil. When the water begins to boil, reduce the heat to low. Cover the lid of the pot and allow its contents to simmer for around 15 minutes. At the end of 15 minutes, remove the pot from the heat. Let it rest in the pot, with the lid covered, for another five minutes. Transfer the cooked quinoa to a large bowl and keep it aside for cooling.

As the quinoa is cooling, let's prepare the balsamic dressing. Take a small bowl. Add the olive oil, honey and balsamic vinegar to it and mix well.

Pour the balsamic dressing over the cooled quinoa and mix well. Add the goat cheese, strawberries, spinach and sunflower seeds to the bowl and mix well. Once the contents of the bowl have mixed well, divide it equally among six serving bowls. Serve immediately.

Raw kale salad with lemon tahini dressing (228 calories per serving)

Yields: 4 servings

Ingredients:

For the Lemon Tahini Dressing (Makes about 1 cup of dressing)

- 1 tablespoon of fat-free Greek Yogurt
- 2 garlic gloves, minced finely
- 3 tablespoons of Tahini
- 1 teaspoon of pepper
- Pinch of salt
- Juice from 2 lemons
- 3 tablespoons of water

For the Salad

- ½ large head of kale
- 1 cup of red onion, finely chopped
- 1 cup of red bell pepper, finely chopped
- ½ cup of carrot, chopped finely
- 1 cup of cherry tomatoes, cut in halves
- ½ cup of cucumber, deseeded and chopped finely
- ¼ cup of chopped almonds
- ¼ cup of reduced-fat shredded parmesan

Instructions:

First, let us prepare the dressing. Add the yogurt, tahini, garlic, pepper and salt to the bowl of a food processor. Pour the lemon juice and water on top of the contents of the food processor. Pulse until the mixture is of a smooth and creamy consistency. Keep the dressing aside.

Now, wash the kale well. Remove the leaves from the stem and chop it coarsely. Place the chopped kale in a large bowl. Add the chopped bell pepper, red onion, cherry tomatoes, cucumber to the bowl and mix well. Add the almonds to the bowl next and mix well.

Pour the dressing on top of the salad and mix well. Once the dressing is evenly distributed, sprinkle the cheese on top of the salad.

Place the bowl in the refrigerator and let it rest for 15 minutes. This should be sufficient time for the flavors to blend well. At the end of fifteen minutes, remove the bowl from the refrigerator. Divide the salad equally among 4 serving bowls. Serve immediately.

Waldorf salad (100 calories per serving)

Yields: 12 servings

Ingredients:

- ½ cup of walnuts, finely chopped
- 4 apples
- 2 cups of celery
- 1 cup of raisins
- ½ cup of non-fat plain yogurt
- 1 teaspoon of sugar
- 2 teaspoons of lemon juice

Instructions:

Preheat the oven to 350 degrees.

Wash the apples well. Peel their skins off and cut them in halves. Remove the cores and the seeds. Cut the apple into smaller pieces and keep aside.

Wash the celery well and cut into smaller pieces.

Arrange the chopped walnuts neatly on a baking sheet. Allow it to bake in the oven for around 12 to 15 minutes. Stir the walnuts occasionally to ensure that they are toasted in a uniform fashion.

Add the toasted walnuts to a big bowl. Add the chopped apples and celery to the bowl and mix well. Next, add the raisins and nuts to the bowl and mix well.

Take another small bowl. Add the lemon juice, sugar and yogurt to the bowl and mix well.

Pour the yogurt dressing on top of the apple mixture and toss lightly.

Place the bowl in the refrigerator and let it rest for 15 minutes. This should be sufficient time for the flavors to blend well. At the end of fifteen minutes, remove the bowl from the refrigerator. Divide the salad equally among 6 serving bowls. Serve immediately.

Barley, corn and bean salad (110 calories per serving)

Yields: 12 servings

Ingredients:

- 1 can of kidney beans, rinsed and drained
- 1 cup of fresh corn
- 2 cups of pearl barley
- 1 large red bell pepper, deseeded and chopped finely
- ¼ cup of thinly sliced green onion
- 1 clove of garlic, finely chopped
- ½ cup of thinly sliced celery
- ¼ cup of fresh lime or lemon juice
- 2 tablespoons of vegetable oil
- 1/8 teaspoon of salt
- ¼ teaspoon of pepper
- Finely chopped fresh cilantro, for garnish
- Water

Instructions:

Take a medium sized saucepan. Pour the water into it. Add the barley to the pan. Bring the water to a boil. Once the water starts boiling, reduce the heat to low. Cover the pan with a lid and cook it covered for around forty five minutes. At the end of forty five minutes, remove the pan from the heat and transfer the cooked barley to a bowl. Add cold water to the bowl and rinse the cooked barley well. Drain the water.

Add the corn, kidney beans, green onion, red bell peppers, celery and garlic to the bowl and mix well. Add the vegetable oil, pepper and salt to the bowl and mix well.

Place the bowl in the refrigerator and cover it with a lid. Let it rest for few hours. This should be sufficient time for the flavors to blend well. At the end of few hours, remove the bowl from the refrigerator. Divide the salad equally among 12 serving bowls. Garnish with the chopped cilantro and serve immediately.

Latin Cabbage slaw (110 calories per serving)

Yields: 6 servings

Ingredients:

- ¼ cup of apple cider vinegar
- 2 tablespoons of agave nectar
- ¼ teaspoon of kosher salt
- ¼ teaspoon of chili powder
- ¼ cup of canola oil
- 4 cups of shredded green cabbage
- Juice from 2 limes or lemons
- ½ cup of red bell pepper, thinly sliced
- ½ cup of green bell pepper, thinly sliced
- 6 to 8 green onions, thinly sliced
- ½ cup of fresh cilantro, chopped coarsely

Instructions:

Take a medium sized bowl. Add the apple cider vinegar, agave nectar, kosher salt, lime or lemon juice, oil and chili powder to it. Whisk well and keep aside.

Take a large bowl. Add the shredded cabbage, sliced red bell pepper, green bell pepper, green onions and cilantro. Mix well.

Pour the dressing on top of the contents of the large bowl. Mix well to ensure that the dressing is evenly distributed. Taste the salad. Add more agave nectar, chili powder, lime juice or a pinch of the salt, if you want more seasonings.

Place the bowl in the refrigerator and let it rest for 15 minutes. This should be sufficient time for the flavors to blend well. At the end of fifteen minutes, remove the bowl from the refrigerator. Divide the salad equally among 6 serving bowls. Serve immediately. This salad will stay good for 2 days, if you keep it refrigerated.

Conclusion

For amazing results on lowering blood pressure and losing weight, adopt a DASH diet for three meals a day including the dessert and snack in between the main meal. You don't need medicine when you can do it the natural way.

Thank you again for buying this book!

I hope the DASH diet recipes in this book will be of great help to you even as you try to lose weight and maintain your blood pressure at a healthy level.

The next step is to adapt a DASH diet today for a healthier you.

Finally, if you enjoyed this book, would you be kind enough to leave a review for this book on Amazon?

Click here to leave a review for this book on Amazon!

Thank you and good luck!